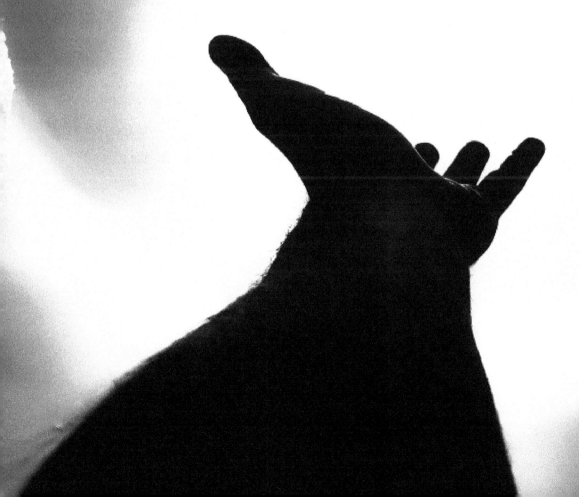

"The greatest treasures are those invisible to the eye, but felt by the heart"

MARYANNE WILLIAMSON

THE WONDER OF IT ALL

"Our intention creates our reality"
– Wayne Dyer

the Programs

GOLD CYCLE

The Gold Frequencies were developed together with the Portuguese clinical director and researcher Nuno Nina, who has applied them to thousands of clients for over 15 years. The Gold Cycle is based on three programs: BALANCE, BEING, and PURE. BALANCE is designed to harmonize the Bioenergetic Field of the physical, BEING the emotional body, while PURE promotes recovery from environmental causes of energetic imbalance. These three programs can be used alternately every day to strengthen your bioenergetic field. The CARE program can be used when you feel your system is particularly challenged.

The recommended usage for each of the programs listed is once daily.

BALANCE
The fine balance of the various bodily systems is very important for our well-being and health. The BALANCE program refers to bioenergetic harmony. It is an ideal program for a deep bioenergetic harmonization of the body's overall energy field.
Duration: 52 minutes

BEING
What the program BALANCE is for the body, BEING is for our soul. It is designed to help you remain centered during life's turmoil.
Duration: 55 minutes

CARE
A weakened Bioenergetic Field is frequently associated with poor health. Strengthen your energy field through proper exercise, healthy nutrition, and pure water, and restoring bioenergetic harmony are all ways of caring for your inner and outer health.
Duration: 46 minutes

ENERGY
Performance needs support. Whether you are a well-trained competitive athlete, a stressed-out manager, or a busy mother, ENERGY increases your ability to respond to life's demands.
Duration: 55 minutes

PURE
The PURE program is the ideal starting point for anyone using the Healy App IMF (Individual Microcurrent Frequency) programs for the first time. It is designed to help your body's energy field recover from the bioenergetic effects of environmental factors.
Duration: 52 minutes

RELAX

RELAX stands for harmonizing your stress response. Stress can be both the result and the cause of imbalances in the mind and body that can undermine your health and wellbeing. Modern life keeps many of us from letting go of our daily sorrows and stress, so support for you in this area can help you restore your sense of balance.

Duration: 55 minutes

RELEASE

There are many different causes of discomfort. In this program, you work systemically to address the energetic source of the discomfort in the Bioenergetic field.

Duration: 46 minutes

PAIN / STIMULATION

Pain can have various causes and is basically a warning signal from the body that something is physically or psychologically wrong. Since pain often affects muscles, joints, the head, organs, or tissue, pain therapy is one of the largest areas in modern medicine. Pain is often a complex entity of physical trauma and trauma memory, tissue acidification, tissue toxicity, cell energy reduction, or lack of regeneration.

Pain has a bilateral effect, which means that information flows in two directions: physical pain influences emotions, and the psyche – conversely, emotions, and the psyche clearly influence pain.

The recommended usage for each of the programs listed is once daily.

CHRONIC PAIN (I)
Relief of chronic pain via the CNS (Central Nervous System)
Duration: 20 minutes

CHRONIC BACK PAIN (II)
Local relief of chronic back pain
Duration: 20 minutes

TOOTH – JAW LOCAL (III)
Local supportive treatment of pain in the mouth area
Duration: 20 minutes

JOINTS LOCAL (IV)
Local relief of joint pain
Duration: 20 minutes

MIGRAINE (V)
Cranial (head side) treatment of migraine
Duration: 20 minutes

INSOMNIA (VI)
Supportive treatment of sleep issues via the CNS (Central Nervous System)
Duration: 20 minutes

DEPRESSION (VII)
Supportive treatment of depressed feelings via the CNS (Central Nervous System)
Duration: 20 minutes

ANXIETY (VIII)
Relief of anxious feelings via the CNS (Central Nervous System)
Duration: 20 minutes

LEARNING

Learning succeeds particularly well when it is fun, easy, and relaxed.

Today, even young adults face big challenges: examination stress, mental strain, grade pressure, social anxiety, and others. This can manifest itself in concentration problems, burnout, compulsive and self-defeating behaviors, lack of motivation, or unpredictable moods.

The learning programs are for harmonizing the Bioenergetic Field, which can support memory, concentration, stress reduction, problem-solving, and creativity.

University and career training students can particularly profit from Healy technology during exam time. Healthy habits can be supported in the Bioenergetic Field as well as learning and concentration.

The recommended usage for each of the programs listed is once daily.

LEARNING SYST.
Harmonization of the Bioenergetic Field for learning activities.
Duration: 57 minutes

LEARNING ACUTE
Specific harmonization of the Bioenergetic Field to support the ability to focus and retain learning.
Duration: 20 minutes

MEMORY
Harmonization of the Bioenergetic Field for knowledge retention.
Duration: 79 minutes

CONCENTRATION SYST.
Harmonization of the Bioenergetic Field for focus and the ability to ignore distraction.
Duration: 57 minutes

CONCENTRATION ACUTE
Specific harmonization of the Bioenergetic Field to enhance focus.
Duration: 20 minutes

EXAM SYST.
Harmonization of the Bioenergetic Field during exam preparation.
Duration: 57 minutes

EXAM ACUTE

Harmonization of the Bioenergetic Field before exams.

Duration: 30 minutes

STRESS SYST.

Harmonization of the Bioenergetic Field for creative power.

Duration: 57 minutes

STRESS ACUTE

Harmonization of the Bioenergetic Field for stress situations.

Duration: 30 minutes

FITNESS

In today's frequently sedentary lifestyles, maintaining fitness is a good means of balance for physical, mental, and emotional wellbeing. Regular physical activity should always be followed by a recovery phase. In addition, it is essential to maintain a healthy, balanced diet rich in nutrients and fiber. Fitness has also characterized by a sense of becoming balanced and centered within ourselves.

It is always important to feel supported and centered, and all the more so during times of stress, burnout, or grief. The Healy Fitness programs have been developed with this basic idea in mind., These programs include the body as well as the mind we strongly believe that a balanced, sustainable and holistic psychophysiological constitution must encompass both of them.

Healy Fitness programs concentrate on the harmonization of the Bioenergetic Field in four essential areas: muscles, performance, weight, and relaxation. This combination is therefore suitable for everyone who enjoys sports and fitness activities.

The recommended usage for each of the programs listed is once daily.

WEIGHT
Harmonization of the bioenergetic field for your body's energy balance. (not a weight-loss program)
Duration: 60 minutes

MUSCLE
Harmonization of the bioenergetic field for recovery.
Duration: 39 minutes

CIRCULATION
Harmonization of the bioenergetic field for demands of exercise.
Duration: 39 minutes

PERFORMANCE
Harmonization of the bioenergetic field that supports your desire to excel.
Duration: 60 minutes

STRENGTH
Harmonization of the bioenergetic field of strained muscles.
Duration: 60 minutes

STAMINA
Harmonization of the bioenergetic field for optimization of the capacity for endurance.
Duration: 60 minutes

REGENERATION

Harmonization of the bioenergetic field to stimulate vitality.

Duration: 57 minutes

DEEP RELAXATION

Harmonization of the bioenergetic field to optimize the relaxation phase.

Duration: 24 minutes

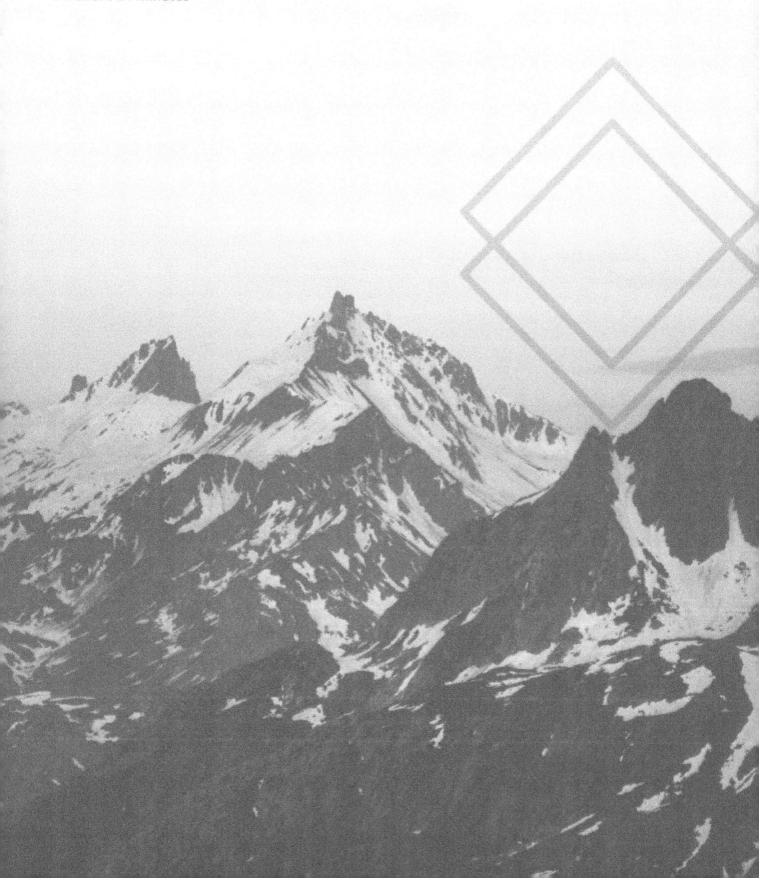

JOB/SLEEP

People leading a stressful working life often feel stuck on a treadmill. They might have been in a situation where they have little opportunity to focus on their own needs and wants. External commitments may seem more important than their inner voice calling for a break or a change of direction. If this call is ignored for too long and if one's own limits are permanently exceeded, the body may adopt a "refusal attitude" that can lead to the deactivation of entire functional areas.

This in turn can lead to prolonged fatigue, exhaustion, sleep disruption, and hypersensitivity to stress.

We spend about one-third of our life sleeping. The need for sleep varies for each individual, but on average it is about 7.5 hours per day. Depending on the age and life situation, 4-12 hours of sleep may be required, in one go or spread over the day. Sleep is vital and serves to regenerate the body and process the impressions of the day. Disturbed sleep can throw us off balance and even make us sick in the long run. Longer lasting sleep disturbances can lead to physical fatigue, health deficits, and a weakening of the immune system. In addition, poor sleep quality can also have a negative emotional effect and strain our psyche.

These programs can provide valuable harmonization of the Bioenergetic Field when leading an active professional life, offering programs for people leading a stressful everyday life.

The recommended usage for each of the programs listed is once daily.

ACTIVATION
Activation of the Bioenergetic Field.
Duration: 57 minutes

POSITIVE THOUGHTS
Energetic orientation towards positive thoughts.
Duration: 45 minutes

BALANCE NERVES
Harmonization of the Bioenergetic Field to promote calmness.
Duration: 60 minutes

FATIGUE
Harmonization of the Bioenergetic Field to promote energetic balance.
Duration: 60 minutes

EXHAUSTION SYST.
Harmonization of the Bioenergetic Field for recreation.
Duration: 60 minutes

SLEEP SYST.

Harmonization of the Bioenergetic Field for optimizing the sleep phase.
Duration: 51 minutes

BED REST

Harmonization of the Bioenergetic Field to promote relaxation.
Duration: 55 minutes

BALANCED SLEEP

Bioenergetic harmonization of the sleep phase.
Duration: 52 minutes

FINE FLOW

Bioenergetic activation through supporting ionic movement in the body
Duration: 20 minutes

MENTAL BALANCE

The mental balance and the subconscious of the human being are complex and host all feelings and thoughts, as well as all mental characteristics and the specific personality traits of a person. The human being is a unity consisting of body, mind, and soul. Thus, as psychosomatics shows, people can have physical complaints caused by mental imbalances.

This influence also works in the opposite direction, so that the body, for example, the intestine, has a great influence on a person's mental balance. If this colloquially called inner or soul life is intact, an individual is balanced and vital. Traumatic experiences are partly unconscious experiences that can reach from the past into the present. They continue to have an effect on the physical as well as the mental and spiritual level, because the trauma has not been processed, integrated, or dissolved.

The recommended usage for each of the programs listed is once daily.

INNER STRENGTH SYST.
Energetic harmonization of self-confidence when you feel uncertain or insecure.
Duration: 51 minutes

EMOTIONAL WELL-BEING
Energetic harmonization when you feel emotionally blocked.
Duration: 51 minutes

FEEL GOOD SYST.
Energetic activation of confidence when you feel down.
Duration: 51 minutes

CONTENTMENT SYST.
Energetic harmonization of the inner sense of self and contentment.
Duration: 60 minutes

CONTENTMENT ACUTE
Supports your sense of inner balance during recovery from nicotine dependence (not a smoking cessation program)
Duration: 20 minutes

INNER UNITY
Energetic harmonization of the sense of psychic wholeness.
Duration: 55 minutes

WELL-BEING SOUL

Energetic harmonization to support you while developing new habits.

Duration: 51 minutes

MENTAL BALANCE ACUTE

Supports positive thinking.

Duration: 20 minutes

BEAUTY / SKIN

The skin forms the physical boundary between the inner and outer world. It is not only a respiratory organ, but also a visible "showpiece" representing beauty, youthfulness, and health. The outer beauty is decisively influenced by the inner beauty, which in turn is influenced by factors such as intestinal health, inner balance, and bliss.

Nuno Nina's experience in harmonizing the Bioenergetic Field for inner balance and relaxation as well as his expertise in defining the appropriate frequencies for harmonizing the Bioenergetic Field of the skin have been integrated into the Healy Beauty programs.

The recommended usage for each of the programs listed is once daily.

INNER BEAUTY
Harmonization of the coherence and expression of the Bioenergetic Field.
Duration: 45 minutes

HAIR
Harmonization of the Bioenergetic Field of the hair.
Duration: 60 minutes

SKIN
Harmonization of the Bioenergetic Field of the skin.
Duration: 60 minutes

AGING
Harmonization of the Bioenergetic Field to relax your expressions.
Duration: 57 minutes

NAILS
Harmonization of the Bioenergetic Field of the nails.
Duration: 42 minutes

SKIN ELASTICITY
Harmonization of the Bioenergetic Field for smooth skin.
Duration: 51 minutes

SUPPORT SKIN LOCAL
Harmonization of the Bioenergetic Field of the skin cells.
Duration: 30 minutes

SUPPORT SKIN SYST.
Harmonization of the skin regeneration in the Bioenergetic Field.
Duration: 60 minutes

SKIN IMPURITY SYST. Harmonization of skin impurities in the Bioenergetic Field.
Duration: 60 minutes

SCARS SYST.
Harmonization of the Bioenergetic Field to balance interference fields.
Duration: 60 minutes

SCARS LOCAL
Harmonization of the Bioenergetic Field of scar tissue.
Duration: 20 minutes

BIOENERGETIC HARMONY 1

Bioenergetic Harmony 1 and Bioenergetic Harmony 2 contain frequency program compilations of the most common applications in everyday life, selected based on the experiences of our users. The use of terms like "immune system" etc. refers to the disharmonies in the Bioenergetic Field that often underlie the symptoms associated with these terms. They are not intended to claim or imply that harmonizing the Bioenergetic Field will have a direct effect on those expressions or will cure, treat, mitigate or prevent any diseases associated with them.,

The recommended usage for each of the programs listed is once daily.

IMMUNE SYSTEM
Harmonization of the bioenergetic field of the energetic defense system.
Duration: 60 minutes

CHILLING
Harmonization of the bioenergetic field of the mucous membranes.
Duration: 51 minutes

HYPERSENSITIVITY
Harmonization of the bioenergetic field in case of overreactions to irritants.
Duration: 60 minutes

EYES
Harmonization of the bioenergetic field of the eyes.
Duration: 65 minutes

HORMONES
Harmonization of the bioenergetic field of the body's "messengers".
Duration: 57 minutes

INTESTINE
Harmonization of the bioenergetic field of the intestine.
Duration: 51 minutes

NERVES
Harmonization of the bioenergetic field to promote relaxation.
Duration: 45 minutes

FLEXIBILITY
Harmonization of the bioenergetic field to ease movement.
Duration: 51 minutes

CIRCULATORY SYSTEM

Harmonization of the bioenergetic field of the circulation.
Duration: 55 minutes

POTENCY

Harmonization of the bioenergetic field of the reproductive organs.
Duration: 60 minutes

MENOPAUSE

Harmonization of the bioenergetic field to help you deal with menopause.
Duration: 66 minutes

MENSTRUATION LOCAL

Harmonization of the bioenergetic field to promote relaxation of the lower abdomen.
Duration: 20 minutes

BIOENEREGETIC HARMONY 2

GASTROINTESTINAL

Harmonization of the bioenergetic field of digestion.

Duration: 60 minutes

BACTERIA

Harmonization of the bioenergetic field of the defense system.

Duration: 60 minutes

TONSILS

Harmonization of the bioenergetic field to reduce feelings of discomfort.

Duration: 60 minutes

LIVER

Harmonization of the bioenergetic field of the liver.

Duration: 52 minutes

FOOD SENSITIVITIES

Harmonization of the bioenergetic field in case of food sensitivities.

Duration: 60 minutes

TOXINS

Harmonization of the bioenergetic field of the excretory processes.

Duration: 60 minutes

HEAD

Harmonization of the bioenergetic field to reduce tension.

Duration: 72 minutes

PROSTATE

Harmonization of the bioenergetic field of the prostate.

Duration: 60 minutes

LUNGS

Harmonization of the bioenergetic field of the lungs.

Duration: 51 minutes

THYROID GLAND

Harmonization of the bioenergetic field of the thyroid gland.

Duration: 60 minutes

JOINTS / BONES

Harmonization of the bioenergetic field of the joints and bones.

Duration: 72 minutes

SCIATICA LOCAL

Harmonization of the bioenergetic field of the sciatic nerve.

Duration: 20 minutes

MERIDIANS 1

Traditional Chinese medicine (TCM) claims that life energy (Qi) flows in channels or meridians. According to this concept, there are twelve main channels and each meridian is assigned to a functional circle (organ system). The corresponding acupuncture points are therefore threaded onto the meridians like pearls on a string. Furthermore, acupuncture points have relationships or connections to organs or parts of organs which the acupuncturist activates by stimulation and thus endeavors to positively influence the state of the organ.

These programs according to the meridian system of Dr. Reinhold Voll are designed to harmonize blockages in the Bioenergetic Field of the individual meridians.

The recommended usage for each of the programs listed is once daily.

ALLERGY MERIDIAN
Harmonization of the bioenergetic field of the allergy meridian.
Duration: 60 minutes

CONNECTIVE TISSUE
Harmonization of the bioenergetic field of the connective tissue meridian.
Duration: 51 minutes

BLADDER
Harmonization of the bioenergetic field of the bladder meridian.
Duration: 51 minutes

LARGE INTESTINE
Harmonization of the bioenergetic field of the large intestine meridian.
Duration: 51 minutes

SMALL INTESTINE
Harmonization of the bioenergetic field of the small intestine meridian.
Duration: 51 minutes

FATTY DEGENERATION
Harmonization of the bioenergetic field of the fatty degeneration meridian.
Duration: 51 minutes

GALL BLADDER
Harmonization of the bioenergetic field of the gall bladder meridian.
Duration: 51 minutes

JOINTS

Harmonization of the bioenergetic field of the joints meridian.

Duration: 51 minutes

SKIN

Harmonization of the bioenergetic field of the skin meridian.

Duration: 51 minutes

HEART

Harmonization of the bioenergetic field of the heart meridian.

Duration: 63 minutes

Traditional Chinese medicine (TCM) claims that life energy (Qi) flows in channels or meridians. According to this concept, there are twelve main channels and each meridian is assigned to a functional circle (organ system). The corresponding acupuncture points are therefore threaded onto the meridians like pearls on a string. Furthermore, acupuncture points have relationships or connections to organs or parts of organs which the acupuncturist activates by stimulation and thus endeavors to positively influence the state of the organ.

These programs according to the meridian system of Dr. Reinhold Voll are designed to harmonize blockages in the Bioenergetic Field of the individual meridians.

The recommended usage for each of the programs listed is once daily.

HORMONAL BALANCE
Harmonization of the bioenergetic field of the hormonal balance meridian.
Duration: 51 minutes

CIRCULATION
Harmonization of the bioenergetic field of the circulation meridian.
Duration: 51 minutes

LIVER
Harmonization of the bioenergetic field of the liver meridian.
Duration: 54 minutes

LUNGS
Harmonization of the bioenergetic field of the lungs meridian.
Duration: 51 minutes

LYMPHATIC SYSTEM
Harmonization of the bioenergetic field of the lymphatic system meridian.
Duration: 51 minutes

STOMACH
Harmonization of the bioenergetic field of the stomach meridian.
Duration: 51 minutes

SPLEEN / PANCREAS
Harmonization of the bioenergetic field of the spleen-pancreas meridian.
Duration: 51 minutes

NERVE MERIDIAN

Harmonization of the bioenergetic field of the nerve meridian.

Duration: 51 minutes

KIDNEY

Harmonization of the bioenergetic field of the kidney meridian.

Duration: 54 minutes

ORGAN MERIDIAN

Harmonization of the bioenergetic field of the organ meridian.

Duration: 54 minutes

CHAKRAS

The chakra system is thousands of years old and references to it can be found in many cultures all over the world. The Hopi, Inca, and Maya cultures, for example, make references to the chakras.

A large part of Asian teachings and religions are based on the principles of the Indian chakra teachings. The influence of the Indian chakra teachings reaches so far that they form the foundation for Buddhism and Hinduism, as well as for various techniques of energy and bodywork, such as Yoga, Tai Chi, Ayurveda, TCM, and spiritual healing.

Furthermore, the spiritual, as well as energy practitioner circles, have adopted these teachings as the basis of many methods of energy and healing work.

The recommended usage for each of the programs listed is once daily.

CROWN CHAKRA
Traditional Theme: Higher Self
Harmonization of the energies of the crown chakra.
Duration: 33 minutes

THIRD EYE CHAKRA
Traditional Theme: Intuition
Harmonization of the energies of the third eye chakra.
Duration: 33 minutes

THROAT CHAKRA
Traditional Theme: Communication
Harmonization of the energies of the throat chakra.
Duration: 33 minutes

HEART CHAKRA
Traditional Theme: Empathy
Harmonization of the energies of the heart chakra.
Duration: 33 minutes

SOLAR PLEXUS CHAKRA
Traditional Theme: Self-Confrdence
Harmonization of the energies of the solar plexus chakra.
Duration: 33 minutes

SACRAL CHAKRA

Traditional Theme: Creativity

Harmonization of the energies of the sacral chakra.

Duration: 33 minutes

ROOT CHAKRA

Traditional Theme: Trust

Harmonization of the energies of the root chakra.

Duration: 33 minutes

BIOENERGETIC DEFENSE

GENERAL PROTECTION
Energetic shielding
Duration: Unlimited

ELECTROSENSITIVITY
Energetic balancing of the tolerance for so-called "electrosmog".
Duration: Unlimited

CELL
Energetic harmonization of the Bioenergetic field of the cell.
Duration: Unlimited

MENTAL
Energetic promotion of clear perceptual capacity.
Duration: Unlimited

SLEEPING
Energetic protection during sleep.
Duration: Unlimited

GEOPATHY
Energetic reduction of sensitivity to interference fields.
Duration: Unlimited

SUBTLE
Energetic protection against external influence.
Duration: Unlimited

PLANETS
Harmonizing the influences of planets
Duration: Unlimited

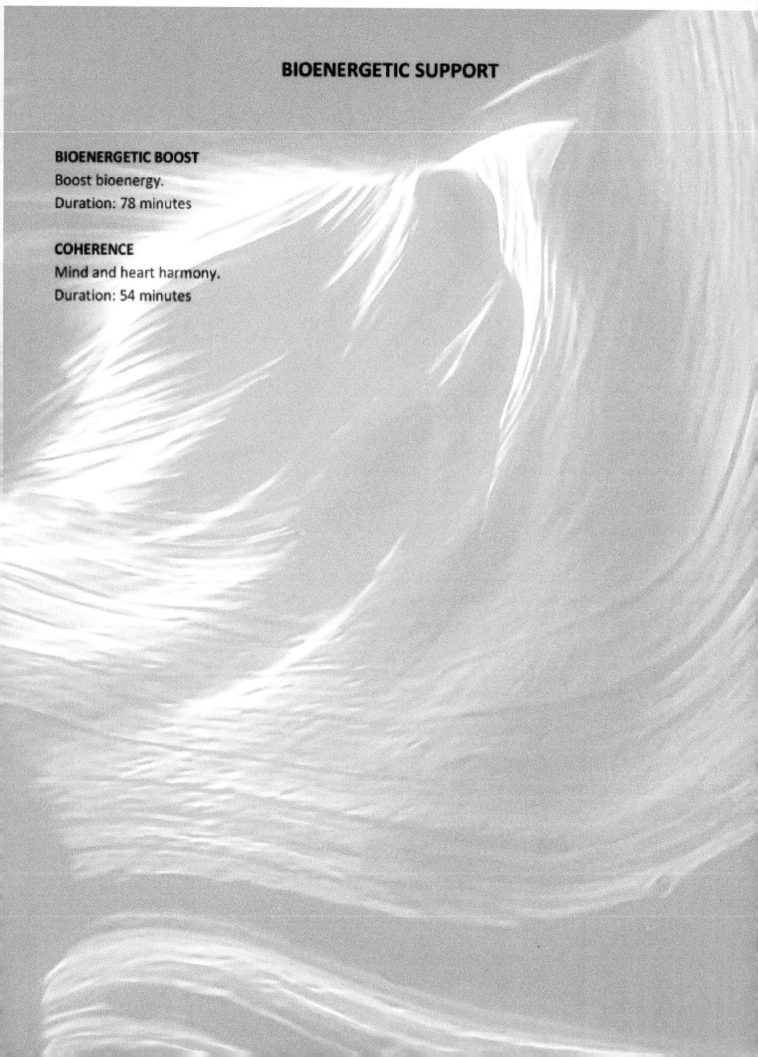

BIOENERGETIC SUPPORT

BIOENERGETIC BOOST
Boost bioenergy.
Duration: 78 minutes

COHERENCE
Mind and heart harmony.
Duration: 54 minutes

BIOENERGETIC VITALISATION

REGENERATION I

Harmonization of the Bioenergetic Field to stimulate vitality first phase.

Duration: 30 minutes

REGENERATION II

Harmonization of the Bioenergetic Field to stimulate vitality second phase

Duration: 30 minutes

REGENERATION III

Harmonization of the Bioenergetic Field to stimulate vitality third phase

Duration: 30 minutes

BONES

Harmonization of the Bioenergetic Field of the bones

Duration: 29 minutes

TISSUE

Harmonization of the Bioenergetic Field of the tissue

Duration: 30 minutes

STABILITY

Harmonization of the Bioenergetic Field for stability

Duration: 16 minutes

HOLISTIC SUPPORT

Harmonization of the Bioenergetic Field for holistic support

Duration: 34 minutes

NERVES

Harmonization of the Bioenergetic Field of the nerves

Duration: 32 minutes

PINEAL GLAND

Harmonization of the Bioenergetic Field of the pineal gland

Duration: 30 minutes

YOUTH

Harmonization of the Bioenergetic Field for optimization of the capacity for activity

Duration: 22 minutes

EPIGENETIC HARMONIZATION

Harmonization of the Bioenergetic Field of the cell epigenetic

Duration: 30 minutes

CELL

Harmonization of the Bioenergetic Field of the cells

Duration: 35 minutes

DEEP CYCLE H

The Deep Cycle programs are in daily use in the Uno Vita – Klinik for Integrert Medisin (Integrated Medicine Clinic) in Oslo, Norway, and many of its clients use them at home too. The Deep Cycle IMF programs are a variation and further development of the popular Nuno Nina Gold Cycle IMF programs and can be beneficially combined with them for harmonizing the Bioenergetic Field. The development of the Deep Cycle IMF programs is the result of Jan Fredrik Poleszynski's experience in microcurrent frequency applications since 2009 and is closely connected to the integrative thinking of Nuno Nina and his Gold Frequencies. The Deep Cycle IMF programs have a special position in applications in the bio- energetic field and are generally more comprehensive than the Gold Cycle IMF programs.

The systemic therapy by Nuno Nina and the Deep Cycle programs belong to alternative medicine and represent a bio-energetic balancing.

In his clinic for integrated medicine in Oslo, Jan Fredrik Poleszynski treats several clients with chronic fatigue or impaired cell metabolism. Clients with chronic health problems use other additional programs, such as CLEAN ALL, along with a more concrete program like DIGEST ALL, if they still have digestive issues after a longer period of applications. If the digestion issues are directly linked to stress, PURE CALM can be helpful for bio-energetic balancing.

SENSITIVE
When: Well suited for sensitive people, including those affected with electro sensitivity.
Affirmation and intention: The environment is my soil.
Duration: 41 minutes

PURE ENERGY
When: The main part of the Pure Energy program is focused on balancing emotions, spiritual balance and supporting wellbeing.
Affirmation and intention: All is energy.
Duration: 62 minutes

ENERGY WORK
When: The main purpose of the Energy Work program is to increase the energetic harmony. It is recommended to use it in the morning.
Affirmation and intention: An abundance of energy is flowing
Duration: 241 minutes

BREATH OF LIFE
When: There are energetic issues associated with lungs and their surrounding organs, including the breast, along with feelings related to weakness and occasional sad feelings.
Body: Lungs and all energetic afflictions in the surrounding area
Affirmation and intention: My breath is a reflection of the breath of the universe
Duration: 52 minutes

CLEAN ALL

When: Appropriate for follow-up after energetic purification as an energetic support for all purification pathways. It is advisable to include this program in a sequence of applications, as any release on any level of the system often causes a need for purification. To release old blockages from the energetic body and mind.

Body: Complete energetic purification of various systems, such as kidneys, lungs, liver, digestive system, lymph, and circulation system

Affirmation and intention: My body is pure, I feel comfortable in it. Duration: 59 minutes

DIGEST ALL

When: Recommended for disharmonies in the Bioenergetic Field of the digestion that blocks further progress. For this program, adhesive electrodes can be used. They should be placed at the level of the ankle on the front side of the foot acupuncture point ST 42.

Body: Intestines, stomach, pancreas, gallbladder

Affirmation and intention: I accept my past, digest and integrate it.

Duration: 48 minutes

GO TO THE ROOTS

When: Only use when the symptoms have subsided and the recovery process has begun. All essential energetic functions should work normally. The energetic causes on the mental level and emotional patterns will now be addressed. This program is suitable as the conclusion of a series of applications.

Body: Intestines, stomach, pancreas, gallbladder

Affirmation and intention: I feed my roots and grow into a strong tree.

Duration: 47 minutes

FREE FLOW

When: To energetically harmonize the Bioenergetic Field of the circulation. It is suitable for use after basic harmonization of the Bioenergetic Field of the kidney and lungs, as well as for general energetic stiffness.

Body: Intestines, stomach, pancreas, gallbladder

Affirmation and intention: My movement, blood flow, and circulation are powerful

Duration: 42 minutes

RENEWAL

When: If energetic harmonization is desired.

Body: Bones, skin, tendons, vessels, nerves, muscles, and DNA

Affirmation and intention: Everything is restored, pain is temporary

Duration: 45 minutes

KIDNEY ALL FEMALE & KIDNEY ALL MALE

When: To harmonize the Bioenergetic Field of the kidneys and harmonize energetic processes that are related to the kidney according to Traditional Chinese Medicine. The acupuncture point K5 to K6 (below the ankle on the inside of the foot) is suitable for electrode placement. K5 to K6 (or SP6) is close to the tibial nerve, which can also be indirectly stimulated.

Caution: Do not use SP6 or K5-K6 stimulation during bleeding, which also includes menstruation.

Body: Kidney, adrenals, bladder, urinary system, ovaries, genitals, prostate and related bio- energetic problems

Affirmation and intention: My energy flows freely

Duration KIDNEY ALL FEMALE: 49 minutes

Duration: KIDNEY ALL MALE: 52 minutes

PURE CALM

When: It should contribute to inner peace, emotional and spiritual balance.

Body: Energetic Muscle relaxation. The other parts of the program are intended to support the non-physical aspects of life

Affirmation and intention: I'm connected to everything

Duration: 39 minutes

DIGITAL NUTRITION MIXTURES 1

BRAIN *(body)*

Vitamin B1, Coenzyme Q10, Vitamin B2, Vitamin B6, Magnesium, Potassium, Sulfur, Cobalt, Zinc, Glycine, Phenylalanine

HAIR *(body)*

Vitamin B12, Vitamin B2, Vitamin B5, Biotin, Vitamin B9, Inositol, Iron, Manganese, Zinc, Copper, Molybdenum, Vitamin B10, Cysteine, Silicon Dioxide, Seleniumium

SKIN *(body)*

Coenzyme Q10, Seleniumium, Silicon Dioxide, Vitamin A, Vitamin B2, Vitamin B3, Vitamin B5, Vitamin B6, Vitamin B7, Vitamin B10, Vitamin D, Potassium, Sulfur, Zinc, Copper, Cysteine, Threonine, Chromium,

HEART *(body)*

Coenzyme Q10, Potassium, Sodium, Chlorine, Calcium, Phosphorus, Magnesium, Molybdenum

HEAD *(body)*

Chlorine, Iron, Vitamin B1, Vitamin B10, Vitamin B12, Vitamin B5, Vitamin B2, Vitamin B6, Coenzyme Q10, Sulfur

GASTROINTESTINAL SYSTEM *(body)*

Magnesium, Molybdenum, Vitamin B1, Copper, Potassium

MUSCLES *(body)*

Phosphorus, Sodium, Carnitine, Calcium, Iron, Isoleucine, Glycine, Chromium, Silicon Dioxide, Chlorine, Vitamin B5, Magnesium

NAILS *(body)*

Iron, Cysteine, Selenium, Vitamin B2, Zinc

NERVES *(body)*

Vitamin B1, Vitamin B6, Vitamin B9, Vitamin B12, Vitamin B3, Isoleucine, Tryptophan, Molybdenum, Alanine, Liothyronine

KIDNEY *(body)*

Vitamin B1, Vitamin B2, Vitamin B5, Vitamin B6, Vitamin B7, Vitamin B9, Vitamin B12, Vitamin C, Vitamin D, Calcium, Iron, Zinc, Copper, Taurine, Selenium, Histidine, Phosphorus, Magnesium, Carnitine, Aspartic Acid, Sodium, Chloride, Potassium, Glutathione

EARS *(body)*

Manganese, Potassium, Zinc, Vitamin E, Vitamin B3

THYROID *(body)*

Iodine, Chromium, Selenium, Phenylalanine

DIGITAL NUTRITION MIXTURES 2

AGE *(metabolism)*

Vitamin A, Vitamin B1, Vitamin B6, Vitamin B8, Vitamin B10, Vitamin B9, Vitamin B12, Vitamin B13, Vitamin C, Vitamin K,

Vitamin D, Coenzyme Q10, Tryptophan, Tyrosine, Citrulline, Calcium, Sulfur, Phosphorus, Copper, Cysteine, Glutathione, Glutamine, Glycine, Serine, Leucine, Valine, Zinc, Iron, Selenium, Magnesium

AMINO ACIDS *(metabolism)*

Valine, Leucine, Threonine, Methionine, Phenylalanine, Tryptophan, Lysine, Histidine, Ornithine- Arginine, Glycine, Alanine, Serine, Cysteine, Tyrosine, Proline, Taurine, Glutamine

ALKALINE POWDER *(metabolism)*

Calcium, Magnesium, Potassium, Zinc, Manganese, Glutamine

CONNECTIVE TISSUE *(metabolism)*

Silicon Dioxide, Manganese, Vitamin C, Glycine, Proline, Threonine

BLOOD *(metabolism)*

Copper, Iron, Molybdenum, Vitamin B12, Vitamin K, Threonine, Calcium, Manganese

WEIGHT *(metabolism)*

Vitamin B2, Vitamin C, Vitamin E, Vitamin D, Iodine, Iron, Calcium, Selenium, Chromium, Carnitine, Leucine, Citrulline, Taurine, 5-HTP, Magnesium, Serotonin

LIVER *(metabolism)*

Vitamin E, Vitamin C, Vitamin A, Vitamin D, Vitamin B1, Vitamin B2, Vitamin B6, Vitamin B10, Vitamin B9, Vitamin B12, Vitamin K, Iron, Zinc, Copper, Selenium, Potassium, Ornithine-Arginine, Aspartic Acid, Citrulline, Glycine, Leucine, Valine, Coenzyme Q10, Taurine, Cystine

MINERALS *(metabolism)*

Sodium, Potassium, Calcium, Magnesium, Phosphorus, Chloride, Sulfur

TRACE ELEMENTS *(metabolism)*

Chromium, Cobalt, Iron, Iodine, Copper, Manganese, Molybdenum, Selenium, Silicon Dioxide, Zinc, Vanadium, Flouride

VEGAN *(metabolism)*

Vitamin A, Vitamin B1, Vitamin B2, Vitamin B6, Vitamin B9, Vitamin B12, Vitamin D, Vitamin C, Iron, Zinc, Calcium, Iodine, Sulfur, Selenium, Carnitine, Taurine, Valine, Lysine, Proline, EPA

VITAMIN B COMPLEX *(metabolism)*

Vitamin B1, Vitamin B2, Vitamin B3, Vitamin B4, Vitamin B5, Vitamin B6, Vitamin B7, Vitamin B8, Vitamin B9, Vitamin B10, Vitamin B12, Vitamin B13, Vitamin B17

HYPOVITAMINOSIS *(metabolism)*

Vitamin B1, Vitamin B2, Vitamin B3, Vitamin B4, Vitamin B5, Vitamin B6, Vitamin B7, Vitamin B8, Vitamin B9, Vitamin B10, Vitamin B12, Vitamin A, Vitamin D, Vitamin E, Vitamin K, Vitamin C

DIGITAL NUTRITION MIXTURES 3 (Detox, Hormonal System, Immune System)

ALCOHOL INTAKE *(detox)*

Vitamin B1, Vitamin B2, Vitamin B3, Vitamin B5, Vitamin B6, Vitamin B9, Vitamin B12, Vitamin E, Vitamin D, Potassium, Selenium, Phosphorus, Manganese, Magnesium, Calcium, Methionine, Molybdenum, Boron, Cysteine, Choline

ANTIOXIDANTS *(detox)*

Vitamin A, Vitamin E, Vitamin C, Vitamin B2, Vitamin B10, Flavonoide, Coenzyme Q10, Selenium, Zinc, Manganese, Copper, Iron, Chromium, Glutathione, Melatonin, Cysteine, Glutamine, Methionine, Taurine

LYMPHATIC SYSTEM *(detox)*

Silicon Dioxide, Potassium, Copper, Zinc, Calcium, Magnesium, Vitamin C, Vitamin B6, Vitamin E, Lysine, Proline, Methionine, EPA, Ornithine-Arginine, Glutathione

MENSTRUATION *(detox)*

Calcium, Magnesium, Manganese, Vitamin B5, Vitamin B6, Vitamin E

SPIRITUALITY *(detox)*

Vitamin B1, Vitamin B3, Vitamin B9, Vitamin B12, Vitamin E, Vitamin D, Vitamin K, Coenzyme Q10, Iron, Selenium, Zinc, Manganese, Flavonoide, Tyrosine, Taurine, Tryptophan, Carnitine, Glycine, Glutamine, EPA, Cysteine, Methionine, Glutathione

TOXINS *(detox)*

Vitamin B1, Vitamin B2, Vitamin B3, Vitamin B5, Vitamin B6, Vitamin B9, Vitamin B12, Vitamin C, Vitamin E, Cholin, Cysteine, Methionine, Glutathione, Glycine, Taurine, Glutamine, Aspartic Acid, Flavonoids, Selenium, Zinc, Copper, Iron, Calcium, Magnesium, Silicon Dioxide

FERTILITY *(hormonal system)*

Coenzyme Q10, Carnitine, Vitamin A, Zinc, Manganese

HORMONAL SYSTEM *(hormonal system)*

Vitamin B6, Vitamin B9, Vitamin B10, Vitamin D, Vitamin E, Sulfur, Zinc, Manganese, Iron, Iodine, Selenium, Calcium, Leucine, Lysine, Phenylalanine, Threonine, Tryptophan, Glutamine, Ornithine- Arginine, Glycine, Proline, Cysteine, Tyrosine, Methionine, Valine, Melatonin, Serotonin, Corticosterone

LIBIDO *(hormonal system)*

Vitamin E, Vitamin A, Zinc, Manganese

ALLERGIES *(immune system)*

Vitamin B3, Vitamin C, Vitamin D, Calcium, Sulfur, Proline, Phytinsäure, Quercetin

IMMUNE SYSTEM *(immune system)*

Vitamin A, Vitamin C, Vitamin E, Cysteine, Liothyronine, Sulfur, Glycine, Threonine, Valine, Arginine, Carnitine, Calcium, Copper, Manganese, Zinc, Cobalt, Molybdenum, Selenium

SECONDARY PLANT SUBSTANCES *(immune system)*

Flavonoide, Carotinoide

DIGITAL NUTRITION MIXTURES 4 - Vitality, Sports, Others

ENERGY *(vitality)*

Vitamin B1, Vitamin B2, Vitamin B5, Vitamin B7, Coenzyme Q10, Iron, Zinc, Selenium

FATIGUE *(vitality)*

Vitamin B1, Vitamin B2, Vitamin B5, Vitamin B7, Vitamin B10, Vitamin B6, Coenzyme Q10, Potassium, Sulfur, Iron, Zinc, Selenium, Molybdenum, Glycine, Alanine, Liothyronine, Methionine, Vitamin B9, Vitamin B12, Vitamin B6, Isoleucine, Chromium, Tryptophan, Copper

EYESIGHT *(vitality)*

Vitamin A, Zinc

SPORTS *(sports)*

Vitamin C, Vitamin D, Vitamin B1, Vitamin B2, Vitamin B6, Vitamin B3, Vitamin B7, Vitamin B9, Vitamin B12, Vitamin B13, Coenzyme Q10, Carnitine, Calcium, Potassium, Sodium, Chloride, Magnesium, Zinc, Iron, Phosphorus, Chromium, Vanadium, Glutamine, Cysteine, Phenylalanine, Threonine, Taurine, Valine, Glycine, Glutathione, Androsterone, Aspartic Acid

MEN *(sports)*

Vitamin C, Vitamin E, Vitamin D, Vitamin B1, Vitamin B2, Vitamin B6, Vitamin B9, Vitamin B12, Magnesium, Calcium, Selenium, Zinc, Boron, Coenzyme Q10, Flavonoide, EPA, Androsterone, Aspartic Acid

REGENERATION *(sports)*

Vitamin C, Vitamin E, Vitamin B6, Vitamin B7, Vitamin B13, Carnitine, Copper, Selenium, Zinc, Iron, Iodine, Magnesium, Potassium, Calcium, Chromium, Methionine, Glutamine, Ornithine- Arginine, Glycine, Histidine, Leucine, Valine, Methionine, Cysteine, Glutathione, Coenzyme Q10

WOMEN *(other)*

Vitamin A, Vitamin C, Vitamin D, Vitamin E, Vitamin K, Vitamin B1, Vitamin B2, Vitamin B6, Vitamin B9, Vitamin B12, Calcium, Iron, Aspartic Acid, Ornithine-Arginine, Zinc, Magnesium, Iodine, Silicon Dioxide, Glucosamine Sulfate, Carnitine, Coenzyme Q10, Flavonoide, EPA

CHILDREN *(other)*

Vitamin A, Vitamin C, Vitamin D, Vitamin E, Vitamin B1, Vitamin B2, Vitamin B5, Vitamin B6, Vitamin B9, Vitamin B12, Iron, Zinc, Magnesium, Manganese, Selenium, Copper, Iodine, Calcium, Potassium, Threonine, Ornithine-Arginine, Tryptophan, EPA

PSYCHE *(other)*

Vitamin B3, Vitamin B5, Vitamin B6, Vitamin B9, Vitamin B10, Vitamin B12, Sulfur, Zinc, Copper, Chromium, Cobalt, Tryptophan, Methionine, Phenylalanine, Glutamine, 5-HTP, Threonine, Glycine, Serotonin, Melatonin

SLEEP *(other)*

Vitamin B3, Tryptophan, Glycine, Glutamine

GROWTH *(other)*

Vitamin A, Vitamin B9, Vitamin B12, Zinc, Manganese, Selenium

WOUNDS *(other)*

Vitamin B1, Vitamin B5, Vitamin B6, Vitamin B9,
Vitamin C, Vitamin E, Potassium, Silicon Dioxide, Zinc, Isoleucine, Threonine

DIGITAL NUTRITION MIXTURES 5 – Sports, Musculoskeletal System, Cardiovascular, Metabolism

BREATH *(sports)*

Vitamin A, Vitamin B6, Vitamin B9, Vitamin B12, Vitamin C, Vitamin E, Vitamin D, Selenium, Zinc, Magnesium, Cysteine, Sulforaphane, EPA, Glutathione

MOTION *(sports)*

Vitamin C, Vitamin E, Vitamin A, Vitamin B1, Vitamin B2, Vitamin B6, Magnesium, Calcium, Iron, Potassium, Zinc, Sodium, Iodine, Copper, Glutathione, EPA, Chromium, Carnitine, Coenzyme Q10, Ornithine -Arginine, Methionine, Glycine

COMPETITION *(sports)*

Carnitine, Glycine, Methionine, Ornithine – Arginine, Glutamine, Magnesium, Potassium, Iron, Coenzyme Q10, Selenium, Vitamin C, Vitamin E, Vitamin B6, Taurine, Sodium, Chloride, EPA

STRUCTURE *(musculoskeletal system)*

Alanine, Glycine, Proline, Valine, Leucine, Lysine, Vitamin C, Zinc, Copper, Iodine, Sodium, Calcium, Potassium, Magnesium

MOBILITY *(musculoskeletal system)*

Vitamin B12, Vitamin B6, Vitamin A, Vitamin C, Vitamin E, Vitamin D, Vitamin B1, Vitamin K, EPA, Glucosamine Sulfate, Silicon Dioxide, Histidine, Cysteine, Magnesium, Calcium, Manganese, Copper, Carnitine, Glycine, Lysine, Proline

ACTIVATION *(musculoskeletal system)*

Vitamin B1, Vitamin B2, Vitamin B12, Vitamin B4, Vitamin B6, Vitamin B9, Vitamin C, Vitamin D, Iron, Magnesium, Coenzyme Q10, Taurine, Carnitine, Glycine, Lysine, Zinc, Tyrosine, Phenylalanine, Tryptophan, Choline, Glutamine, Glutathione

REDUCTION *(cardiovascular)*

Vitamin A, Vitamin C, Vitamin K, Vitamin E, Vitamin D, Vitamin B1, Vitamin B2, Vitamin B3, Vitamin B5, Vitamin B6, Vitamin B7, Vitamin B9, Vitamin B12, Glutathione, Magnesium, Cobalt, Copper, Chromium, EPA, Coenzyme Q10, Flavonoide, Ornithine – Arginine, Taurine, Glycine, Glutamine, Lysine

EXERTION *(cardiovascular)*

Coenzyme Q10, Ornithine – Arginine, Vitamin B6, Carnitine, Taurine, Vitamin C, Vitamin B12, Vitamin B9, Magnesium, Vitamin D, EPA, Flavonoids, Potassium, Glutathione

CIRCULATION *(cardiovascular)*

Vitamin A, Vitamin B12, Vitamin B9, Vitamin D, Iron, Ornithine – Arginine, Glutamine, Selenium, Zinc, Calcium, Potassium, Phosphorus, Flavonoids, EPA, Glutathione, Histidine, Magnesium, EPA, Coenzyme Q10, Taurine, Lysine

RIGIDITY *(metabolism)*

Iron, Phenylalanine, Cysteine, Vitamin C, Vitamin B10, Valine, Proline, Vitamin D, Copper, Vitamin E, Flavonoids, Magnesium, Coenzyme Q10, Carnitine, Phosphorus, Glycine, Zinc

LIFESTYLE *(metabolism)*

Vitamin B3, Vitamin B9, Vitamin B6, Vitamin B8, Vitamin B12, Vitamin C, Vitamin D, Vitamin E, Glutathione, EPA, Chromium, Coenzyme Q10, Carnitine, Selenium, Zinc, Copper, Magnesium

ENERGETIC *(metabolism)*

Vitamin B1, Vitamin B2, Iron, Selenium, Zinc, Vitamin B12, Vitamin B3, Vitamin B9, Manganese, Copper, Vitamin C, Vitamin A, Vitamin D, Vitamin K, Methionine, Histidine, Magnesium, Coenzyme Q10, Carnitine, EPA

DIGITAL NUTRITION MIXTURES 6 (METABOLISM, HORMONAL SYSTEM, OTHER)

TISSUE *(metabolism)*

Vitamin C, Vitamin D, Coenzyme Q10, Vitamin B5, Vitamin B10, Vitamin B12, Selenium, Proline, Cortisone, Tryptophan, Copper, EPA, Flavonoide, Potassium

BIO INFORMATION *(metabolism)*

Vitamin A, Vitamin E, Vitamin B2, Vitamin B6, Vitamin B7, Vitamin B9, Vitamin B12, Methionine, Choline, EPA, Glycine, Magnesium, Selenium, Zinc, Iron, Copper, Manganese, Calcium, Chromium, Glutathione

COMFORT *(metabolism)*

Vitamin D, Vitamin C, Vitamin E, Vitamin K, Vitamin B9, Chromium, Magnesium, Coenzyme Q10, EPA, Zinc, Vanadium, Taurine, Ornithine – Arginine, Carnosine, Carnitine, Cysteine, Glycine, Sulforaphane, Flavonoide, Corticosterone

EXHAUSTION *(hormonal system)*

Vitamin B1, Vitamin B2, Vitamin B3, Vitamin B5, Vitamin B6, Vitamin B7, Vitamin B9, Vitamin B12, Sodium, EPA, Glutamine, Taurine, Corticosterone, Vitamin C, Cortisone, Magnesium, Tryptophan, Ornithine – Arginine, Potassium

MENOPAUSE *(hormonal system)*

Vitamin C, Vitamin E, Vitamin D, Vitamin K, Vitamin B2, Vitamin B1, Vitamin B9, Vitamin B12, Vitamin B6, Flavonoids, Selenium, Magnesium, Zinc, Calcium, Ornithine – Arginine, Tryptophan, EPA

PASSION *(hormonal system)*

Vitamin B6, Vitamin B9, Vitamin B12, Vitamin D, Selenium, Zinc, Glutathione, Coenzyme Q10, Carnitine, Aspartic Acid

BALANCE *(other)*

Vitamin B6, Vitamin B9, Vitamin B12, Vitamin D, Vitamin E, Iron, Selenium, Zinc, Magnesium, Glutathione, Flavonoide, Glutamine, Ornithine – Arginine, Aspartic Acid

RELIEF *(other)*

Vitamin B2, Vitamin B5, Vitamin B1, Vitamin B7, Vitamin B3, Vitamin B9, Vitamin B10, Vitamin B12, Selenium, Ornithine – Arginine, Vitamin C, Vitamin D, Zinc, Glycine, Magnesium, Vitamin E, Tryptophan, EPA

JOY OF LIFE *(other)*

5-HTP, Serotonin, Tryptophan, Vitamin B3, Vitamin B5, Vitamin B6, Vitamin B9, Vitamin B10, Vitamin B12, Phenylalanine, Cobalt, Androsterone, Glutamine, Copper, Sulfur, EPA, Citrulline, Chromium, Methionine, Zinc, Thyroxine

RECREATION *(other)*

Tryptophan, Serotonin, Magnesium, Vitamin B1, Vitamin B2, Vitamin B3, Vitamin B6, Vitamin B12, Vitamin D, Vitamin C, Selenium, Melatonin, Coenzyme Q10, Manganese, Molybdenum

REST *(other)*

Tryptophan, Serotonin, Melatonin, Glycine, Ornithine -Arginine, Vitamin D, Vitamin B3, Vitamin B5, Vitamin B6, Vitamin B9, Vitamin B10, Vitamin B12, Iron, Zinc, Copper, Selenium, Magnesium, Methionine, Phenylalanine

TEETH *(other)*

Vanadium, Coenzyme Q10, Vitamin K, Vitamin C, Vitamin B6, Glucosamine Sulfate, Phosphorus, Vitamin B12, Manganese, Copper, Vitamin B9, Vitamin E, Vitamin A, Vitamin D, Calcium

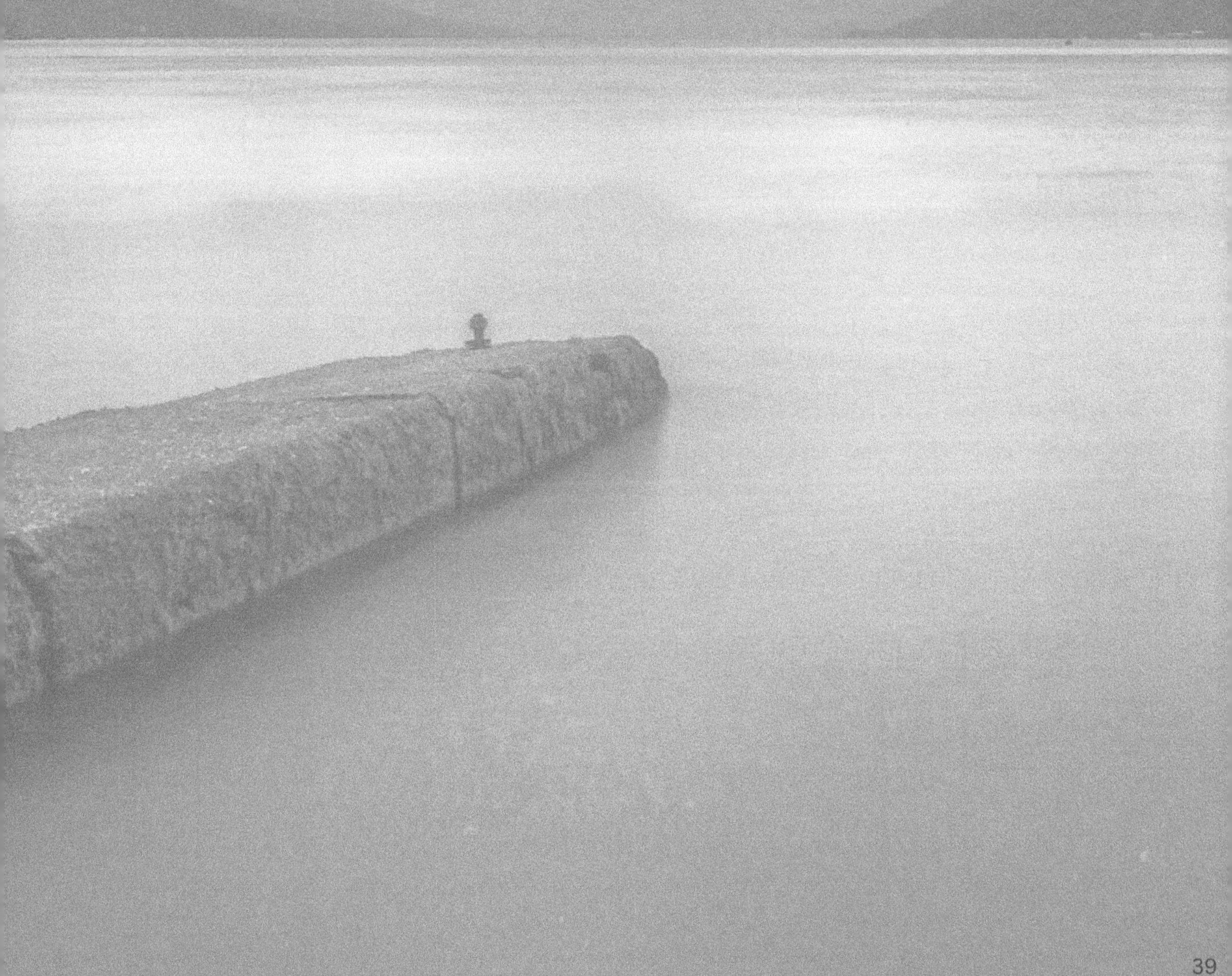

POWER OF THREE

We are living in times of individual and collective energetic traumatization and polarization on many levels, its causes and consequences touching the physical, mental, emotional, and spiritual aspects of our human nature. The controversies and consequences of global events have created a need for bioenergetic and subtle harmonization and balancing.

The Power of Three Healy program group is our response to the energetic and informational bifurcation point (or branching situation) perceived and experienced by many among us. It is based on the ancient system of three natural energetic forces, as expressed in the bioenergies of Ayurveda.

Three groups, each containing three programs Combining a systematic analysis of current collective processes and classical universal frequencies, the Power of Three programs are designed for a special 9-week application protocol.

Run programs by group, one program at a time, once a day on Mondays, Wednesdays, and Fridays and then proceed to next program in group until all 3 programs (3 days & 3 weeks worth are complete), then proceed to next group and repeat.

GROUP 1 - Universal Frequencies
The classical frequencies
1. Classical Physical
2. Classical Energetic
3. Zapper Protocol

GROUP 2 - Digital Ayurveda
The soothing power and ancient wisdom of digital Ayurveda. Mix and match, or choose one of two according to your personal Ayurvedic type!
1. Kapha
2. Pitta
3. Vata

GROUP 3 - Bioenergetic Rebalance
For use in especially difficult energetic times!

1. Conflict Balance
2. Defense Support
3. Friendly Flora

EXPERT HEALY PROGRAMS

Expert programs were once only accessible through a private consultation with a TimeWaver Therapist with access to a TimeWaver machine. Now, you can purchase custom and expert programs to use with your Healy from the comfort of your home.

Meet Derek

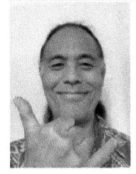

Derek is a TimeWaver Therapist and has also been a Massage Therapist since 2000 (and still enjoys working on clients!). Everything changed for him in 2009 when his wife returned home from a Bioresonance session and immediately told Derek that they needed the same system. Unfortunately, that particular system would require Derek to learn Russian so they did more research to try to find a device that would be easier to understand with support in English. In 2010 they started with a system from the UK and it was just two years later that they found TimeWaver. Derek started with TimeWaver Med and then added TimeWaver Frequency in 2017 after attending the TimeWaver World Conference in Germany. And, now, naturally, Derek and his wife have added Healy to their family of TimeWaver devices and are successfully working with clients all over the world. Derek has a wealth of information at his fingertips and his experience and continued education ensure that he is able to create the best custom programs to meet the needs of his clients.

https://dereknakamura.com/shop/

Meet Brid Hanlon

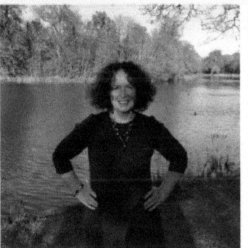

Teacher, Homeopath, Healer and Energy Practitioner
25 YEARS EXPERIENCE IN THE FIELDS OF HEALING AND PERSONAL DEVELOPMENT

OVER 15 YEARS PRACTICING AS A TEACHER, QUALIFIED COUNSELLOR AND HOMEOPATH

8 YEARS AS A RESPECTED AND EXPERIENCED ENERGY THERAPIST
With over 20 years experience in the fields of Health, Healing and Spiritual growth, I'm a respected and highly experienced Energy practitioner, working successfully with clients all over the world.
After qualifying as a Science teacher in my 20's, I went on to train first as a Person-Centered Counsellor and then as a Homeopath, before being introduced to the Quantum healing technology. I felt an instant excitement on discovering the combing of Science and Spirituality for the benefit of mankind.

https://www.bridhanlon.com/programs

Reference Charts

GOLD

Order No.	Program name	Technology	Duration	Frequency
1	Pure	IMF	52 min	1 x Daily
2	Care	IMF	46 min	1 x Daily
3	Balance	IMF	52 min	1 x Daily
4	Being	IMF	55 min	1 x Daily
5	Energy	IMF	55 min	1 x Daily
6	Relax	IMF	55 min	1 x Daily
7	Release	IMF	46 min	1 x Daily

LEARNING

Order No.	Program name	Technology	Duration	Frequency
1	Learning syst.	IMF	57 min	1 x Daily
2	Learning acute	MC	20 min	1 x Daily
3	Memory	IMF	79 min	1 x Daily
4	Concentration syst.	IMF	57 min	1 x Daily
5	Concentration acute	MC	20 min	1 x Daily
6	Exam syst.	IMF	57 min	1 x Daily
7	Exam acute	MC	30 min	1 x Daily
8	Stress syst.	IMF	57 min	1 x Daily
9	Stress acute	MC	30 min	1 x Daily

FITNESS

Order No.	Program name	Technology	Duration	Frequency
1	Weight	IMF	60 min	1 x Daily
2	Muscle	IMF	39 min	1 x Daily
3	Circulation	IMF	30 min	1 x Daily
4	Performance	IMF	60 min	1 x Daily
5	Strength	IMF	60 min	1 x Daily
6	Stamina	IMF	60 min	1 x Daily
7	Regeneration	IMF	57 min	1 x Daily
8	Deep relaxation	IMF	24 min	1 x Daily

JOB

Order No.	Program name	Technology	Duration	Frequency
1	Activation	IMF	57 min	1 x Daily
2	Positive Thoughts	IMF	45 min	1 x Daily
3	Balance Nerves	IMF	60 min	1 x Daily
4	Fatigue	IMF	60 min	1 x Daily
5	Exhaustion syst.	IMF	60 min	1 x Daily
6	Exhaustion acute	MC	20 min	1 x Daily
7	Extreme Stress	IMF	60 min	1 x Daily

SLEEP

Order No.	Program name	Technology	Duration	Frequency
1	Sleep syst.	IMF	51 min	1 x Daily
2	Bed rest	IMF	55 min	1 x Daily
3	Balanced Sleep	IMF	52 min	1 x Daily
4	Fine flow	MC	20 min	1 x Daily

BEAUTY

Order No.	Program name	Technology	Duration	Frequency
1	Inner beauty	IMF	45 min	1 x Daily
2	Hair	IMF	60 min	1 x Daily
3	Skin	IMF	60 min	1 x Daily
4	Aging	IMF	57 min	1 x Daily
5	Nails	IMF	42 min	1 x Daily
6	Skin elasticity	IMF	51 min	1 x Daily

SKIN

Order No.	Program name	Technology	Duration	Frequency
1	Support Skin local	MC	30 min	1 x Daily
2	Support Skin syst.	IMF	60 min	1 x Daily
3	Skin impurity syst.	IMF	60 min	1 x Daily
4	Scars syst.	IMF	60 min	1 x Daily
5	Scars local	MC	20 min	1 x Daily

MENTAL BALANCE

Order No.	Program name	Technology	Duration	Frequency
1	Inner Strength syst.	IMF	51 min	1 x Daily
2	Emotional Well-being	IMF	51 min	1 x Daily
3	Feel good syst.	IMF	51 min	1 x Daily
4	Contentment syst.	IMF	60 min	1 x Daily
5	Contentment acute	MC	20 min	1 x Daily
6	Inner Unity	IMF	55 min	1 x Daily
7	Well-being Soul	IMF	51 min	1 x Daily
8	Mental balance acute	MC	20 min	1 x Daily

BIOENERGETIC HARMONY 1

Order No.	Program name	Technology	Duration	Frequency
1	Immune system	IMF	60 min	1 x Daily
2	Chilling	IMF	51 min	1 x Daily
3	Hypersensitivity	IMF	60 min	1 x Daily
4	Eyes	IMF	65 min	1 x Daily
5	Hormones	IMF	57 min	1 x Daily
6	Intestine	IMF	51 min	1 x Daily
7	Nerves	IMF	45 min	1 x Daily
8	Flexibility	IMF	51 min	1 x Daily
9	Circulatory System	IMF	55 min	1 x Daily
10	Potency	IMF	60 min	1 x Daily
11	Menopause	IMF	66 min	1 x Daily
12	Menstruation local	MC	20 min	1 x Daily

BIOENERGETIC HARMONY 2

Order No.	Program name	Technology	Duration	Frequency
1	Gastrointestinal	IMF	60 min	1 x Daily
2	Bacteria	IMF	60 min	1 x Daily
3	Tonsils	IMF	60 min	1 x Daily
4	Liver	IMF	52 min	1 x Daily
5	Food Sensitivities	IMF	60 min	1 x Daily
6	Toxins	IMF	60 min	1 x Daily
7	Head	IMF	72 min	1 x Daily
8	Prostate	IMF	60 min	1 x Daily
9	Lung	IMF	51 min	1 x Daily
10	Thyroid gland	IMF	60 min	1 x Daily
11	Joints-Bones	IMF	72 min	1 x Daily
12	Sciatica local	MC	20 min	1 x Daily

MERIDIANS 1

Order No.	Program name	Technology	Duration	Frequency
1	Allergy Meridian	IMF	60 min	1 x Daily
2	Connective Tissue	IMF	51 min	1 x Daily
3	Bladder	IMF	51 min	1 x Daily
4	Large intestine	IMF	51 min	1 x Daily
5	Small intestine	IMF	51 min	1 x Daily
6	Fatty degeneration	IMF	51 min	1 x Daily
7	Gallbladder	IMF	51 min	1 x Daily
8	Joints	IMF	51 min	1 x Daily
9	Skin	IMF	51 min	1 x Daily
10	Heart	IMF	63 min	1 x Daily

DEEP CYCLE H

Order No.	Program name	Technology	Duration	Frequency
1	First Application	IMF	42 min	1 x Daily
2	Second Application	IMF	42 min	1 x Daily
3	Third Application	IMF	39 min	1 x Daily
4	Breath of life	IMF	52 min	1 x Daily
5	Clean all	IMF	59 min	1 x Daily
6	Digest all	IMF	48 min	1 x Daily
7	Go to the roots	IMF	47 min	1 x Daily
8	Free flow	IMF	42 min	1 x Daily
9	Renewal	IMF	45 min	1 x Daily
10	Kidney all female	IMF	49 min	1 x Daily
11	Kidney all male	IMF	52 min	1 x Daily
12	Pure calm	IMF	39 min	1 x Daily

DIGITAL NUTRITION MIXTURES 1

Order No.	Program name	Technology	Duration	Frequency
1	Brain	IMF	60 min	1 x Daily
2	Hair	IMF	60 min	1 x Daily
3	Skin	IMF	87 min	1 x Daily
4	Heart	IMF	33 min	1 x Daily
5	Head	IMF	42 min	1 x Daily
6	Gastrointestinal System	IMF	33 min	1 x Daily
7	Muscles	IMF	60 min	1 x Daily
8	Nails	IMF	24 min	1 x Daily
9	Nerves	IMF	51 min	1 x Daily
10	Kidney	IMF	60 min	1 x Daily
11	Ears	IMF	33 min	1 x Daily
12	Thyroid	IMF	24 min	1 x Daily

DEEP CYCLE H

Order No.	Program name	Technology	Duration	Frequency

DEEP CYCLE H

Order No.	Program name	Technology	Duration	Frequency
1	First Application	IMF	42 min	1 x Daily
2	Second Application	IMF	42 min	1 x Daily
3	Third Application	IMF	39 min	1 x Daily
4	Breath of life	IMF	52 min	1 x Daily
5	Clean all	IMF	59 min	1 x Daily
6	Digest all	IMF	48 min	1 x Daily
7	Go to the roots	IMF	47 min	1 x Daily
8	Free flow	IMF	42 min	1 x Daily
9	Renewal	IMF	45 min	1 x Daily
10	Kidney all female	IMF	49 min	1 x Daily
11	Kidney all male	IMF	52 min	1 x Daily
12	Pure calm	IMF	39 min	1 x Daily

DIGITAL NUTRITION MIXTURES 1

Order No.	Program name	Technology	Duration	Frequency
1	Brain	IMF	60 min	1 x Daily
2	Hair	IMF	60 min	1 x Daily
3	Skin	IMF	87 min	1 x Daily
4	Heart	IMF	33 min	1 x Daily
5	Head	IMF	42 min	1 x Daily
6	Gastrointestinal System	IMF	33 min	1 x Daily
7	Muscles	IMF	60 min	1 x Daily
8	Nails	IMF	24 min	1 x Daily
9	Nerves	IMF	51 min	1 x Daily
10	Kidney	IMF	60 min	1 x Daily
11	Ears	IMF	33 min	1 x Daily
12	Thyroid	IMF	24 min	1 x Daily

DIGITAL NUTRITION MIXTURES 2

Order No.	Program name	Technology	Duration	Frequency
1	Age	IMF	60 min	1 x Daily
2	Amino Acids	IMF	60 min	1 x Daily
3	Alkaline Powder	IMF	24 min	1 x Daily
4	Connective Tissue	IMF	24 min	1 x Daily
5	Blood	IMF	33 min	1 x Daily
6	Weight	IMF	51 min	1 x Daily
7	Liver	IMF	69 min	1 x Daily
8	Minerals	IMF	24 min	1 x Daily
9	Trace Elements	IMF	51 min	1 x Daily
10	Vegan	IMF	87 min	1 x Daily
11	Vitamin B Complex	IMF	33 min	1 x Daily
12	Hypovitaminosis	IMF	60 min	1 x Daily

DIGITAL NUTRITION MIXTURES 3

Order No.	Program name	Technology	Duration	Frequency
1	Alcohol Intake	IMF	69 min	1 x Daily
2	Antioxidants	IMF	78 min	1 x Daily
3	Lymphatic System	IMF	60 min	1 x Daily
4	Menstruation	IMF	24 min	1 x Daily
5	Spirituality	IMF	69 min	1 x Daily
6	Toxins	IMF	69 min	1 x Daily
7	Fertility	IMF	33 min	1 x Daily
8	Hormonal System	IMF	69 min	1 x Daily
9	Libido	IMF	24 min	1 x Daily
10	Allergies	IMF	42 min	1 x Daily
11	Immune System	IMF	69 min	1 x Daily
12	2ry Plant Substances	IMF	51 min	1 x Daily

DIGITAL NUTRITION MIXTURES 4

Order No.	Program name	Technology	Duration	Frequency
1	Energy	IMF	42 min	1 x Daily
2	Fatigue	IMF	96 min	1 x Daily
3	Eyesight	IMF	15 min	1 x Daily
4	Sports	IMF	69 min	1 x Daily
5	Men	IMF	78 min	1 x Daily
6	Regeneration	IMF	51 min	1 x Daily
7	Women	IMF	96 min	1 x Daily
8	Children	IMF	78 min	1 x Daily
9	Psyche	IMF	87 min	1 x Daily
10	Sleep	IMF	24 min	1 x Daily
11	Growth	IMF	24 min	1 x Daily
12	Wounds	IMF	42 min	1 x Daily

DIGITAL NUTRITION MIXTURES 5

Order No.	Program name	Technology	Duration	Frequency
1	Breath	IMF	60 min	1 x Daily
2	Motion	IMF	69 min	1 x Daily
3	Competition	IMF	60 min	1 x Daily
4	Structure	IMF	51 min	1 x Daily
5	Mobility	IMF	78 min	1 x Daily
6	Activation	IMF	78 min	1 x Daily
7	Reduction	IMF	105 min	1 x Daily
8	Exertion	IMF	60 min	1 x Daily
9	Circulation	IMF	78 min	1 x Daily
10	Rigidity	IMF	69 min	1 x Daily
11	Lifestyle	IMF	69 min	1 x Daily
12	Energetic	IMF	78 min	1 x Daily

DIGITAL NUTRITION MIXTURES 6

Order No.	Program name	Technology	Duration	Frequency
1	Tissue	IMF	60 min	1 x Daily
2	Bioinformation	IMF	69 min	1 x Daily
3	Comfort	IMF	87 min	1 x Daily
4	Exhaustion	IMF	60 min	1 x Daily
5	Menopause	IMF	78 min	1 x Daily
6	Passion	IMF	42 min	1 x Daily
7	Balance	IMF	60 min	1 x Daily
8	Relief	IMF	69 min	1 x Daily
9	Joy of Life	IMF	69 min	1 x Daily
10	Recreation	IMF	60 min	1 x Daily
11	Rest	IMF	69 min	1 x Daily
12	Teeth	IMF	60 min	1 x Daily

BIOENERGETIC VITALIZATION PROGRAMS

Order No.	Program name	Technology	Duration	Frequency
1	Regeneration I	IMF	30 min	1 x Daily
2	Regeneration II	IMF	30 min	1 x Daily
3	Regeneration III	IMF	30 min	1 x Daily
4	Bones	IMF	29 min	1 x Daily
5	Tissue	IMF	30 min	1 x Daily
6	Stability	IMF	16 min	1 x Daily
7	Holistic Support	IMF	34 min	1 x Daily
8	Nerves	IMF	32 min	1 x Daily
9	Pineal Gland	IMF	30 min	1 x Daily
10	Youth	IMF	22 min	1 x Daily
11	Epigenetic Harmonization	IMF	30 min	1 x Daily
12	Cell	IMF	35 min	1 x Daily

HEALY ANIMAL PROGRAMS

Order No.	Program name	Technology	Duration	Frequency
1	Eyes	IMF	36 min	1 x Daily
2	Irritant Reactions	IMF	70 min	1 x Daily
3	Hormones	IMF	52 min	1 x Daily
4	Suffering	IMF	52 min	1 x Daily
5	Hypersensitivity	IMF	66 min	1 x Daily
6	Microbiota	IMF	43 min	1 x Daily
7	Rest	IMF	52 min	1 x Daily
8	Cleaning	IMF	52 min	1 x Daily
9	Emotions	IMF	52 min	1 x Daily
10	Power	IMF	52 min	1 x Daily
11	Defense System	IMF	52 min	1 x Daily
12	Joints	IMF	69 min	1 x Daily

WELLBEING

Order No.	Program name	Technology	Duration	Frequency
1	Body	IMF	42 min	1 x Daily
2	Mind	IMF	66 min	1 x Daily
3	Spirit	IMF	66 min	1 x Daily

BIOENERGETIC REBALANCE

Order No.	Program name	Technology	Duration	Frequency
1	Conflict Balance	IMF	54 min	1 x Daily
2	Defense Support	IMF	66 min	1 x Daily
3	Friendly Flora	IMF	66 min	1 x Daily

Natural Cycle

Our life is profoundly influenced by the phases of the moon, the sun and the earth. The frequencies of these celestial bodies determine our bodies, our emotions and perhaps our destiny since the moment of our birth.

But most of us today are leading lives that are moving too fast and causing us to drift away from our natural rhythms. Our body and our mind are sensing these conflicts and many of us experience physical and emotional imbalances.

With the Healy Natural Cycle program group, we can address these challenges by bringing our lives back into alignment with the natural cycles and flow. The Healy Natural Cycle programs contain completely new frequencies, developed and compiled by Nuno Nina, the creator of the Healy Gold Cycle.

The application of the Natural Cycle program must begin on so-called trigger dates (e.g. a change of seasons, an equinox, etc.), when ideal energetic conditions occur in the solar and lunar cycles. At the beginning it is also necessary to determine the organ meridian with which the application should be started. These calculations are conveniently and automatically performed by the HealAdvisor Natural Cycle module, which also reminds the user at the right time for the application when the organ of a particular meridian is active.

Drinking a glass of pure water 30 and 15 minutes prior to the meridian activation program and 15 minutes afterwards will optimally prepare you to use the frequency programs.

In the first weeks of a Natural Cycle, the daily stabilization program is applied. When the stabilizing effect becomes noticeable (easy and refreshed waking up, no problems with bowel movements, timely and easy falling asleep), you switch to the stabilizing program according to the solar cycle. The HealAdvisor Natural Cycle module adjusts this automatically as well.

Likewise, the HealAdvisor Natural Cycle module determines the respective change to the next organ on the Organ Clock; the application takes place each Tuesday and Friday. If the predetermined time for an organ falls within the usual sleeping time, you can skip this session.

Natural Cycle should also be terminated on a trigger date as soon as you feel that you are in harmony with your natural cycle. The calculation of this date is also performed by the HealAdvisor Natural Cycle module. You can start a Natural Cycle protocol again on each trigger date; Nuno Nina recommends repeating it at least twice a year.

Activation Programs

Order No.	Program name	Meridian	Technology	Duration	Frequency
1	3AM-5AM	Lung	IMF	18 min	1 x Daily
2	5AM-7AM	Large Intestine	IMF	18 min	1 x Daily
3	7AM-9AM	Stomach	IMF	18 min	1 x Daily
4	9AM-11AM	Spleen/Pancreas	IMF	18 min	1 x Daily
5	11AM-1PM	Heart	IMF	18 min	1 x Daily
6	1PM-3PM	Small Intestine	IMF	18 min	1 x Daily
7	3PM-5PM	Bladder	IMF	18 min	1 x Daily
8	5PM-7PM	Kidneys	IMF	18 min	1 x Daily
9	7PM-9PM	Pericardium	IMF	18 min	1 x Daily
10	9PM-11PM	Triple Heater	IMF	18 min	1 x Daily
11	11PM-1AM	Gallbladder	IMF	18 min	1 x Daily
12	1AM-3AM	Liver	IMF	18 min	1 x Daily

IMF = Individualized Microcurrent Frequency

Stabilization Programs

Order No.	Program name	Technology	Duration	Frequency
1	Stabilization Daily	IMF	30 min	1 x Daily
2	Stabilization Solar	IMF	30 min	1 x Daily

Program name	Description
03:00-05:00 寅	The Lung meridian is called the "Master of Qi", meaning that it can balance the flow of biological energy and breath in the whole body. It supports the cells as they engage in the energetic exchange of taking in oxygen and releasing waste. The time of regeneration for this important qi modulating meridian is between 3am and 5am. The distribution of qi and ying allows a good lymphatic and energetic flow that happens in the middle of the night when the body is in a very passive or Yin state.
05:00-07:00 卯	The Large Intestine meridian is called the "Water Purifier" since it supports elimination of waste during the day. The large intestine regulates the health of skin, joints and mucosae and regenerates every morning between 5am and 7am. This particular time is very important to rebalance our microbiome and redistribute fluids that will be then eliminated during the day or reabsorbed as hydration.
07:00-09:00 辰	The Stomach meridian is also called the "Great Granary" or grain storage due to its connection with ingested food. It is not only very important to balance digestion, but also supports good sight and eye coordination as well as alertness. The stomach needs to regenerate every morning between 7am and 9am and if well reactivated, it produces enough yang energy to maintain a good body temperature.

Program name	Description
09:00-11:00 巳	The Spleen meridian relates to Yi or "Thought and Memory" and is traditionally associated with assimilation. It plays a role in regulating GuQi or digestive energy, allowing a long-lasting energy supply for the day. The spleen energy is regenerated every day between 9am to 11am. During this time, it is important to allow the energy to flow from the inside to the outside and not vice versa, therefore heavy meals are to be avoided.
11:00-13:00 午	The Heart meridian is considered the body's "Emperor Spirit", the source of consciousness and pure self. The typical state of vacuity dear to the Taoists and Buddhists is historically represented by the empty resonant heart, devoid of stress and passion. The opportunity to empty the heart and brain and favor the transit of energy to the digestive organs is every day between 11am and 1pm. This short break for the brain allows the Heart meridian to promote balance of cognitive and energetic functions.
13:00-15:00 未	The Small Intestine meridian is the seat of "Fire" and digestive energy. It is in the small intestine that the energy for attention and concentration is produced. During this part of the day the Yang Qi has an increased opportunity to circulate in order to better assimilate food and transform it into GuQi or the energy from food and drinks. The regeneration time for the Small Intestine meridian is every day between 1pm to 3pm.
15:00-17:00 申	The Bladder meridian is thought to balance both the output of fluids and the external flow of energy in the nerves. The Bladder meridian in fact produces the largest distribution of qi along the spine and from the head to the toes. The regeneration time for the Bladder meridian is every day between 3pm to 5pm.
17:00-19:00 酉	The Kidney meridian is called the "Root of Life", as water is its element and the most vital component of life and youth. It is the storage of dense energy called Jing, the type of less-flowing energy that constitutes glands and tissues. A loss of Jing is visible through a lower quality of hair, bones and teeth. Between 5pm and 7pm the Kidney meridian can be calmed through the use of juices, activated water or a warm non-caffeinated beverage.
19:00-21:00 戌	The Pericardium meridian supports the microcirculation of qi through the body's vascular system. Due to the daily chrono-biorhythm, the effect of the qi in the periphery begins to travel towards the inner organs at 7pm, thus allowing for an inner energetic nourishment of dense organs.
21:00-23:00 亥	The Triple Heater meridian is comparable to the metabolism in the western view. A healthy triple heater helps maintain a normal temperature and regulate a good balance between O_2 and CO_2 through breathing. The Triple Heater meridian reduces its functions between 9pm and 11pm. A typical sign of the need to recuperate is when you yawn during this 2-hour period.
23:00-01:00 子	The Gallbladder meridian is called the "General" and thought to be the organ of focused energy. It is related to brain function, magnetic energy (from iron metabolism) and willpower. It is thought to be related to energetically balanced eyes and reflexes. The regeneration time for the Gallbladder meridian is between 11pm and 1am.
01:00-03:00 丑	The Liver meridian is the organ of "Life and Energy" and needs a restful night's sleep to recover. The liver is hosting both the Wei Qi (defensive energy) and the blood. Both get purified during the night around 1am and 3am. The Liver meridian also controls the healthy qi of tendons and blood circulation in the eyes and head.

HEALY
DATABASES

ALASKAN GEM ELIXIRS

AQUAMARINE

Indications: repetitive thoughts; overstimulated from studying, worrying, and circular thinking; having difficulty letting go of thoughts and shifting into a meditative state of mind; not present for others because of preoccupation with mental activities.

Healing Qualities: brings a calm, quiet clarity to an overactive mental body; increases the ability to achieve a neutral, serene state of mind; helps create a mental oasis of cool, clear receptivity.

AVENTURINE

Indications: lacking stamina and fortitude; wanting to quit when faced with obstacles, such as one's own limiting belief systems; fearful when facing the unknown; afraid to take risks in order to take the next step in life.

Healing Qualities: strengthens the central vertical axis which stabilizes us during expansion experiences; helps us move into and through new experiences with grace, stamina, and perseverance; good for spiritual trailblazers and pioneers.

AZURITE

Indications: ungrounded communication; communicating from the head rather than through the body; struggling to communicate, straining to push words out; becoming physically depleted when speaking, teaching, or channeling information from non-physical sources.

Healing Qualities: helps us ground our communication; opens and strengthens the connection between the feminine Earth forces and the 5th chakra; helps us communicate with vitality, authenticity, and gentleness.

BLACK TOURMALINE

Indications: environmental toxicity; oversensitive to computers, fluorescent lights, and other sources of electromagnetic pollution; detoxing on the physical, emotional, or mental level in an unbalanced way.

Healing Qualities: a precision tool for the release of toxic energy from the mind, emotions, and physical body; helps us exchange old unwanted energies being held in the auric field for fresh, clean, neutral energy from nature.

BLOODSTONE (AKA – HELIOTROPE)

Indications: energetic stagnation and constipation; weak circulation of physical and emotional energy in the lower chakras and organs of the body; tendency to express emotional negativity; lacking emotional sensitivity and sympathy towards others.

Healing Qualities: strengthens one's connection to the Earth; brings a stronger flow of Earth energy into the 1st and 2nd chakras; stimulates the release of emotional energies that have been stuck in the lower chakras; rebalances these energy centers after trauma or emotional upset.

BRAZILIAN AMETHYST

Indications: over-identification with the gross, material aspects of life; separation from the spiritual realm; weak connection to one's higher self; resistance to bringing the spiritual into the physical.

Healing Qualities: transmutes energy from lower to higher vibratory frequencies; helps to lift energy from an overly material state; helps one sense and experience one's unique spiritual identity in the body.

BRAZILIAN QUARTZ

Indications: tiredness, fatigue, low energy; weak energetic connection to the Earth; toxic or inharmonious energies in the aura; feeling out of touch with one or more aspects of self (physical, emotional, mental, spiritual), as though they were operating in different time zones; chakra out of alignment with each other.

Healing Qualities: the essence of cleansing white light; energizes and synchronizes the subtle bodies, the chakras, and the physical body with the Earth's natural vibration.

CARNELIAN

Indications: burnout, fatigue, low energy during the day; giving in order to receive; a weak sense of personal identity; addicted to helping others; seeking validation and energy from others rather than from within.

Healing Qualities: increases the etheric body's ability to access pranic energy; energizes and clears the nadirs (the energetic interface between the etheric body and the meridians), allowing a greater flow of energy to the meridians.

CHRYSOCOLLA

Indications: unresolved feelings of grief; heart closed down because of past experiences of loss; feeling a need to guard the heart against attack from others; believing that having an open heart will result in being hurt or wounded again; heart not energetically connected to the Earth.

Healing Qualities: opens, softens, and expands the inner dimensions of the heart chakra; helps us release tension and armoring around giving and receiving love; increases flexibility in the mind and body to allow the vibration of love to flow.

CHRYSOPRASE

Indications: alienation; not feeling at home on the planet or comfortable in nature; loving others but not the Earth; a weak connection between the heart chakra and the Earth.

Healing Qualities: brings the heart chakra into harmonious union with the green energy frequency of the planet; synchronizes the subtle bodies with the heart energy of the Earth; helps us accept the Earth as our home.

CITRINE

Indications: mental confusion and distortion; lack of mental clarity and concentration; mental forces dominating the physical and emotional aspects of life; difficulty determining what is in one's highest good; closed to higher sources of wisdom and inner knowing.

Healing Qualities: harmonizes the mental body with higher spiritual laws; increases access to Divine intelligence; amplifies qualities of concentration, centering, and rational mind.

COVELLITE

Indications: *feeling unprotected and vulnerable; too easily stimulated by the energies of others, regardless of their intent; unsure of one's boundaries; unable to claim one's own space; feeling challenged by the environment.*

Healing Qualities: *brings strength, clarity, and definition to the auric field; acts as a protective filter that encourages us to relax energetically, thereby enhancing our natural ability to receive love and support from our environment.*

DIAMOND

Indications: *life experience characterized by struggle; lack of clarity about the future; acting from a confused sense of what one is supposed to do; inability to make commitments; attached to personal will, to how "I" want it to be.*

Healing Qualities: *brings clarity to the 6th chakra; harmonizes Divine and personal will; helps us activate personal will in its highest form; strengthens our ability to act in alignment with our Divine purpose.*

EMERALD

Indications: *fear of not being good enough to deserve being on the planet; weak or abstract connection to the feminine principle and to the Divine Mother; blocking the experience of love in the physical body because of fear; feeling unloved and cut off from one's center.*

Healing Qualities: *a universal heart cleanser and balancer; helps us contact the energies of the Divine Mother and the Divine Feminine; gently coaxes the heart to open to a greater experience of love in the physical body.*

FLUORITE

Indications: *congestion, constriction, or stagnation of energy on any or all levels; rigidity, inflexibility; difficulty manifesting thoughts into action; hard to move one's focus from one area to another.*

Healing Qualities: *the "break up" elixir; increases the circulation of energy in the physical body by breaking up blockages in the etheric body; promotes flexibility on all levels.*

FLUORITE COMBO

Indications: *lacking focus or a clear sense of priorities when dealing with diverse issues that are all coming up to be healed at the same time; feeling out of synch with one's inner processes; a movement of energy between the etheric body and the physical body is not harmonious or synchronized.*

Healing Qualities: *synchronizes movement between the etheric and physical bodies; fine tunes our focus so that we can deal with multiple issues in a healing process with precision, balance, and a clear sense of priorities.*

GOLD

Indications: *low self-esteem; a weak sense of personal identity; little or no confidence in one's ability to create; weak or uninspired masculine energies; difficulty manifesting wants and needs into physical reality; comparing one's accomplishments to others.*

Healing Qualities: helps us access and express the highest aspects of our personal identity; brings strength and balance to the 3rd chakra; helps us tap into our inner truth, joy, and wisdom as sources for our creative power.

GREEN JASPER

Indications: ungrounded; lack of communication with the Earth; energy blocked in the lower chakras; an inconsistent and uneven flow of sexual energy resulting from the shock and trauma of sexual abuse.

Healing Qualities: reconnects body rhythms with the Earth's rhythm when there has been a disruption to the natural flow; helps us connect to the wild feminine; restores earthly sensuality and healthy sexuality.

HEMATITE

Indications: unable to maintain one's boundaries while witnessing a highly charged emotional experience; getting swept away by other people's negative feelings; emotionally codependent; difficulty containing one's own emotional energy, especially in group dynamics.

Healing Qualities: strengthens energetic boundaries in the emotional body; promotes emotional independence rather than codependence; helps us maintain a state of compassionate detachment while witnessing intense emotions in others; helps us boundary our own emotions in a responsible way.

HERKIMER DIAMOND

Indications: cloudy or undeveloped psychic vision; low energy; unable to remember dreams or having confusing dreams full of chaotic imagery; difficulty bringing information from dream symbols into conscious understanding.

Healing Qualities: a highly developed transmitter of white light; promotes clarity of vision; stimulates healing on all levels; facilitates clarity during the dream state; brings balance and focus to the 6th chakra.

JADEITE JADE

Indications: agitated, upset; easily pulled out of center by intense experiences; attached to drama; makes things harder or more involved than they need to be unable to accept the way things are in the moment.

Healing Qualities: a vibration of peace, balance, and timeless simplicity; helps us stay centered in the moment with an awareness and acceptance of our true essence.

KUNZITE

Indications: feelings of guilt and embarrassment concerning one's past actions; out of touch with one's angelic presence; lack of awareness of the angelic love, guidance, and support that is available; heart closed to the flow of spiritual love coming into the body.

Healing Qualities: opens the heart to an awareness of one's angelic presence; helps one experience the spiritual love of the angelic kingdom and integrate it into the physical body.

LAPIS LAZULI

Indications: unable to hear or understand guidance and information from higher sources; difficulty communicating clearly with others, especially about the information that one has received from these sources; overwhelmed by the amount of information coming in.

Healing Qualities: opens and clears channels of communication in the 5th chakra; amplifies the ability to hear and understand information from physical and nonphysical sources at the same time; clears confusion between hearing and knowing.

MALACHITE

Indications: weak energetic connection to the physical world; forward movement in life held up because of a lack of grounding; physical, emotional, mental, and spiritual aspects of self- working at cross-purposes with each other.

Healing Qualities: the primary grounding essence in our system; helps align the physical, emotional, mental, and spiritual levels of our being in a grounded and cohesive way; supports the unity of one's being in all circumstances.

MOLDAVITE

Indications: caught up in the dualities of here or there, now or then; going out of the body for information rather than staying present to receive it; feeling separate and out of touch, especially with the higher self.

Healing Qualities: connectedness; an energetic window into a universal perspective; helps us stay present in the moment while accessing what we need from the higher realms to express our earthly potential.

MONTANA RHODOCHROSITE

Indications: heart closed down after an abrupt loss or separation from a partner or loved one; feeling unsafe in the heart and wanting to escape into one's thoughts; fearful of powerful emotions; unable to process emotions fully in the heart.

Healing Qualities: brings strength and solidity to the 4th chakra; clears confusion and chaos from the heart; clarifies intent and promotes courageous, heart-centered action.

MOONSTONE

Indications: heightened psychic sensitivity during menstruation; touchy, edgy, overreactive; emotional energy blocked and difficult to express in a clear way; lack of sensitivity and intuitive awareness in men and women; hard-edged persona.

Healing Qualities: cleanses and circulates energy in the emotional body; increases feminine energy aspects of receptivity and intuition in women and men; balances and focuses the psychic forces during menses.

OPAL

Indications: burned out; insomnia from overuse of the mental forces; tiredness that is not helped by sleep; excessive use of the fire element; depletion of certain energy frequencies in the chakras and subtle bodies; vital energy reserves used up; emotional exhaustion.

Healing Qualities: rejuvenates spent emotional and mental forces and counteracts the depletion of color frequencies in the aura; feeds all subtle bodies with a full spectrum of luminous colors; replenishes our creative energies.

ORANGE CALCITE

Indications: *sadness; depression of unknown origin; lack of joy in daily life; lethargy; feeling weighed down with no creative spark; unable to see the positive side of everyday situations; greatly affected by seasonal fluctuations of sunlight and darkness.*

Healing Qualities: *dispels darkness and grief; amplifies the body's ability to assimilate light at the cellular level; uplifting, energizing, and warming.*

PEARL

Indications: *irritated by one's problems and difficulties, especially those manifesting in the physical body in a painful way; lacking understanding and compassion for one's healing process.*

Healing Qualities: *promotes the release of layers of irritation in the mental and emotional bodies that manifest in the physical body as hardness and inflexibility; helps one turn antagonism for oneself or one's illness into awareness and acceptance.*

PERIDOT

Indications: *trepidation, fear, or insecurity during the beginning phase of any new experience; projections of failure when attempting to learn or do something new; feeling unprotected in that space where the known has fallen away and the new has not yet become manifest.*

Healing Qualities: *the stone of new beginnings; stabilizes the subtle bodies and the heart chakra during the incubation period of new creative projects; helps us initiate new cycles of learning and experience without fear.*

PYRITE

Indications: *easily influenced by others, especially members of one's peer group; unable to make decisions or stand up for oneself; involved in relationships that are not in one's highest good; tension and instability from not being true to oneself.*

Healing Qualities: *helps us build an energetic foundation in life-based on our highest personal truth; strengthens the sense of self, especially with regard to group dynamics and peer pressure; helps us solidify and honor our true values.*

RHODOCHROSITE

Indications: *deep trauma and emotional pain in the heart; unable to make intimate connections with others; shut down emotionally or sexually as a result of being abused; feeling cut off and alienated from the physical world.*

Healing Qualities: *increases energy, balance, and stability in the heart chakra and in the physical body; brings a balance of nurturing Earth energy to the heart chakra after an experience of deep healing and transformation.*

RHODOLITE GARNET

Indications: *emotionally and energetically disconnected from parts of the body that are in pain or have been injured or operated on; parts of the body won't heal or return to their normal level of function after injury or trauma; poor circulation in certain areas of the body.*

Healing Qualities: increases our ability to inhabit the physical body; helps us reconnect energetically with parts of the body that have been injured or traumatized; rebuilds the web of etheric energy in areas disrupted by accident or injury.

ROSE QUARTZ

Indications: pain held in the heart from traumatic events in one's past; heart closed down because of not being nurtured as a child; difficulty initiating and maintaining intimate contact with others; inner child not receiving nurturing energy from the adult; lack of compassion for oneself and others.

Healing Qualities: opens, softens, and soothes the heart; helps one connect to and nurture the inner child; harmonizes the heart forces so an individual is able to maintain emotional intimacy with oneself and others.

RUBY

Indications: unresolved survival issues blocking energy flow between the Earth and the 1st chakra; constipation of energies in the lower chakras and organs of the body; ambivalence about being present in the physical body; tendency to disconnect from the body during times of chaos and upheaval.

Healing Qualities: energizes and balances the 1st chakra and supports the ability to ground spiritual energy completely into the physical body; increases the upward flow of nurturing Earth energy to all chakras and improves circulation throughout the body.

RUTILE QUARTZ

Indications: overwhelmed by the amount of energy and information coming in from non- physical sources; distortion, confusion, and/or lack of focus and clarity during mediation or attunement; unable to understand or integrate information and guidance from the higher self.

Healing Qualities: promotes precision alignment with higher sources of energy and inspiration; helps us physically anchor the ability to access, synthesize, and communicate information from other dimensions.

SAPPHIRE

Indications: feeling unsupported for being on the Earth; unaware of life purpose; lack of inspiration and commitment; feeling out of touch and out of place; unwilling or unable to take responsibility for why one has incarnated.

Healing Qualities: strengthens devotion and commitment to Divine purpose; promotes loyalty and responsibility to one's true work on the planet; helps us connect to the energetic support we need to do what we came here to do.

SAPPHIRE/RUBY

Indications: weak body/soul connection; lack of alignment between spiritual and physical bodies due to past injury or debilitating disease; difficulty integrating awareness of life purpose into practical, heart-centered action.

Healing Qualities: for balancing spirituality with physical ability; enables us to gently integrate higher purpose into a physical reality and receive physical nurturing through the fulfillment of Divine responsibilities.

SCEPTER AMETHYST

Indications: lacking spiritual perseverance; unable to take an active stand for what one believes in; in a position of authority but lacking in spiritual leadership qualities; one's experience of the spiritual realm is abstract rather than direct.

Healing Qualities: opens and prepares the 7th chakra to receive energy from the higher chakras; helps us activate our highest potential through the embodiment of a new core of spiritual identity, authority, and leadership.

SMOKY QUARTZ

Indications: ungrounded; agitated, disassociated from the physical body; body feels out of synch with the surrounding environment; detoxification happening at too rapid a pace for the physical body to keep up with; jet lag.

Healing Qualities: grounding and calming; regulates and stabilizes the detoxification of unwanted energies from the physical, emotional, and mental bodies; synchronizes body energy with Earth energy.

SPECTROLITE

Indications: seeing with the eyes, but not with the heart; a low creative spark; unable to sense the deeper meaning of life's events; cloudy, dark, or outdated perspective on life; tendency to see the negative in each situation.

Healing Qualities: bathes and nourishes the entire energy system with full-spectrum light; refreshes and renews our perspective; helps us again see the magnificent in the mundane, and the Divine in the ordinary.

STAR SAPPHIRE

Indications: lacking trust in the universe; difficulty making the right choices and connections in life; over concern for the smallest details of one's process; unable to connect energetically with information about one's higher purpose.

Healing Qualities: promotes trust in the universe; helps us focus our awareness on what is necessary for the soul's progression in life; supports the formation of energetic connections with others that promote the realization of our life goals.

SUGILITE

Indications: living with a highly refined or intellectual concept of what the spiritual realm must be like, rather than a grounded, physically embodied understanding of what it is; believing that one must go outside of oneself to truly experience spiritual support.

Healing Qualities: brings depth and a physical richness to our spiritual lives; helps us physically manifest a warmer, more feminine quality of spirituality; promotes an easy acceptance of guidance and support from the spiritual realms.

TIGER'S EYE

Indications: losing a sense of self-identity when dealing with powerful emotions, whether generated by the self or by others; reacting rather than responding; often angry or jealous; strongly affected by the energy of others; always taking things personally.

Healing Qualities: for self-empowerment; strengthens the energetic boundaries between our true nature and our emotional experiences; helps us maintain a strong sense of self-identity when dealing with powerful emotions such as anger, fear, and jealousy.

TOPAZ

Indications: unable to take decisive action that supports one's true self; a confused sense of personal identity; trying to connect to others for energy in inappropriate ways; identifying more with others than with the self.

Healing Qualities: clears energy blockages in the 3rd chakra; helps us tap into appropriate sources of universal energy; strengthens the ability to act decisively from a clear sense of personal identity.

TURQUOISE

Indications: lack of reverence for the Earth; no gratitude for nature's gifts; too busy to honor the sacredness of life; taking without asking or giving something back; living a life without a soul.

Healing Qualities: attunes the energy field to the ancient wisdom and sacredness inherent in all of life; cleanses and deepens our connection to the soul of the Earth; helps us live a life of simplicity with gratitude and reverence for all.

WATERMELON TOURMALINE

Indications: disharmony between the masculine and feminine aspects of the self; lack of balance between giving and receiving; difficulty expressing love for others or receiving love from others.

Healing Qualities: balances the universal polarities of yin and yang; helps us establish equality between the magnetic and dynamic (giving and receiving) qualities of love; brings the green, physical, Earth frequency into harmony with the pink, spiritual angelic qualities of love.

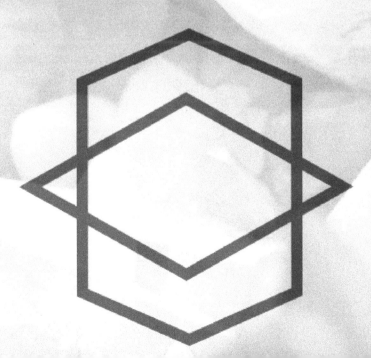

AUSTRALIAN BUSH FLOWERS

Australian Bush Flowers is one of the most comprehensive databases available in the HEALY RESONANCE and HEALY PROFESSIONAL devices one of the reasons why these are Healy World's most popular models.

ALPINE MINT BUSH *(mental and emotional exhaustion)*

This Essence works on the mental and emotional levels. It is for people who work in healing, health administration, or situations where there is a great deal of care for others. These caregivers can be in danger of burning out or becoming disillusioned; they can reach a point of tiredness and feel their life has lost its joy.

Negative Condition: *Mental and emotional exhaustion; lack of joy, and weight of responsibility of caregivers*

Positive Outcome: *Revitalization, joy, renewal*

ANGELSWORD *(spiritual discernment)*

This Essence is for reaching one's own spiritual truth by cutting through any confusion or misinformation. Taking this essence allows access and retrieval of previously developed gifts from past lives. Angelsword protects from outside influences and entities so one can receive clear information from one's Higher Self without interference. Angelsword releases any energies that entered while the aura was open.

Negative Condition: *Interference with a true spiritual connection to Higher Self; spiritually possessed; spiritual confusion*

Positive Outcome: *Spiritual discernment; accessing gifts from past lifetimes; release of negatively held psychic energies; clear spiritual communication*

AUTUMN LEAVES *(releasing the physical plane)*

This Essence allows one to hear, see, and feel communication from the other side and be open to that guidance and communication. It emphasizes the sense of letting go and moving on in a very profound way. The leaves themselves are collected from a sacred area, in autumn, at the exact moment of their release from the trees. This Essence will ease the transition of the passing over from the physical plane to the spiritual world.

Negative Condition: *Difficulties in the transition of passing over from the physical plane to the spiritual world*

Positive Outcome: *Letting go and moving on; increase awareness and communication with loved ones in the spiritual world*

BANKSIA ROBUR *(disheartened, frustrated)*

This Essence addresses temporary loss of drive and enthusiasm due to burnout, disappointment, or frustration. This is for people who are normally very dynamic. When added to bathwater this will assist in washing away negativity.

Negative Condition: *Disheartened; lethargic; frustrated*

Positive Outcome: *Enjoyment of life; enthusiasm; interest in life*

BAUHINIA *(reluctant to change)*

This Essence is for embracing new concepts and ideas. There may be some hesitation or reluctance, initially, in coming to terms with these. It can also help when there is a person who is annoying or whom you dislike.

Negative Condition: *Resistance to change; rigidity; reluctance*

Positive Outcome: *Acceptance; open-mindedness*

BILLY GOAT PLUM (shame, self-loathing)

This Essence is for feelings of shame, self-disgust, and self-loathing. For those people who feel revolted and dirty about sex and feel unclean afterward. It can also be for feelings of revulsion about other physical aspects such as acne, eczema, a large nose, etc.

Negative Condition: Shame; inability to accept the physical self; physical loathing

Positive Outcome: Sexual pleasure and enjoyment; acceptance of self and one's physical body; open- mindedness

BLACK-EYED SUSAN (constant striving, impatience)

This Essence is for people who are impatient or always "on the go". These people are continually rushing, and their lives are always overflowing with commitments. This Essence enables these people to slow down, to find calmness and inner guidance.

Negative Condition: Impatience; "on the go"; over-committed; constant striving

Positive Outcome: Ability to turn inward and be still; slowing down; inner peace

BLUEBELL (closed heart, fear of lack)

This Essence helps to open the heart. It is for those who feel cut-off from their feelings. The emotion is there but is held within. They are subconsciously afraid to express it for they fear their feelings of love, joy, etc. are f,nite or not renewable. They operate from a subconscious fear that there is just not enough and that if they let go of what they have, they will not survive. This fear can often be marked by a controlling, rigid, and forthright manner.

Negative Condition: Closed; fear of lack; greed; rigidity

Positive Outcome: Opens the heart; belief in abundance; universal trust; joyful sharing; unconditional love

BOAB (releasing family patterns)

This Essence is one of the most powerful of all the Bush Essences and has brought about profound change. Boab clears negative emotional and mental family patterns that are passed on from generation to generation. Boab can access and clear those core patterns and all the related ensuing beliefs. This Essence is very beneficial in helping those who have had experiences of abuse or prejudice from others. It will also help clear the negative lines of karma between people.

Negative Condition: Enmeshment in negative family patterns; for recipients of abuse and prejudice

Positive Outcome: Personal freedom by releasing family patterns; clearing of other, non-family, negative Karmic connections

BORONIA (revolving obsessions)

This Essence is for revolving obsessions – thoughts, events, things, or ideas which are stuck. It leads to clarity and focus. It combines well with Bottlebrush for breaking habits and addictions and for dealing with an ended relationship when there is pining for the other person. This Essence also enhances focus for creative visualization.

Negative Condition: Obsessive thoughts; pining; broken-hearted

Positive Outcome: Clarity; serenity; creative visualization

BOTTLEBRUSH (overwhelmed by major change)

This Essence helps people move through major life changes and the overwhelm that often goes with those changes, especially in retirement, menopause, adolescence or death, etc. Bottlebrush is an excellent remedy for pregnant women and new mothers who feel inadequate. It will help throughout pregnancy until after the birth and will assist with bonding between the mother and child. It is excellent for healing unresolved mother issues.

Negative Condition: Unresolved mother issues; overwhelmed by major life changes – old age, adolescence, parenthood, pregnancy, approaching death

Positive Outcome: Serenity and calm; ability to cope and move on; mother-child bonding

BUSH FUCHSIA *(access intuition and trust)*

This Essence assists with problem-solving and improves one's access to intuition – it helps a person to trust their own "gut" feelings. Bush Fuchsia allows for balance between the logical/rational and the intuitive/creative. It will give people courage and clarity in public speaking as well as the ability to speak out about their own convictions.

Negative Condition: Switched-off; nervousness about public speaking; ignoring "gut" feelings; clumsy

Positive Outcome: Courage to speak-out; clarity; in tough with intuition; integration of information; integration of male and female aspects

BUSH GARDENIA *(renew passion in a relationship)*

This Essence is for renewing passion and interest in relationships. It helps draw together those who are moving away from one another, busy in their own world (career, life, etc.). It is not only for romantic relationships but also for family relationships.

Negative Condition: Stale relationships; self-interest; unaware

Positive Outcome: Passion; renews interest in a partner; improves communication

BUSH IRIS *(opening to the spiritual)*

This Essence was one of the first Essences to be prepared. It helps to open people up to their spirituality and to access the doorway to their higher perceptions. It allows the trinity to flow into a person and is an excellent remedy to give someone who has just started the medication of "conscious" spiritual growth.

Negative Condition: Fear of death; materialism; atheism; physical excess; avarice

Positive Outcome: Awakening of spirituality; acceptance of death as a transition state; clearing blocks in the base chakra and trust center.

CHRISTMAS BELL *(lack of abundance)*

This Essence assists one with mastery of the physical plane and with stewardship of one's possessions. It also helps one to manifest their desired outcomes and is extremely beneficial for anyone experiencing a sense of lack. Christmas Bell, operating at a deep spiritual level, helps one to also realize that the most important things in life are not physical and not to be distracted by having their time and energy consumed in the pursuit of these worldly things.

Negative Condition: Lack of abundance; a sense of lack; poor stewardship of one's possessions

Positive Outcome: Helps one to manifest their desired outcome; assists one with mastery of the physical plane

CROWEA *(continually worrying)*

This Essence is for people who are feeling "not quite right" with themselves and are just a little out of balance. It is excellent for people not sure of what it is they are feeling and is great for those who always have something to worry about, without having specific fears.

Negative Condition: Continual worrying; a sense of being "not quite right"

Positive Outcome: Peace and calm; balances and centers the individual; clarity of one's feelings

DAGGER HAKEA *(resentment, holding grudges)*

This Essence is for people who feel resentment and bitterness and hold grudges against those with whom they have been very close (e.g. family members and old lovers). This resentment is often not openly displayed.

Negative Condition: Resentment; bitterness towards close family, friends, lovers

Positive Outcome: Forgiveness; open expression of feelings

DOG ROSE *(apprehension, fear of others)*

This Essence is for treating fears, niggling little fears, not terror. It is also for shy, insecure, timid, nervous people.

Negative Condition: Fearful; shy; insecure; apprehensive of others; niggling fears

Positive Outcome: Confidence; belief in self; courage; ability to embrace life more fully

DOG ROSE OF THE WILD FORCES *(fear of losing control)*

This Essence deals with fear. It is taken when a person has a fear of losing control, when the emotions they are feeling within themselves or immediately around them are just so intense there is a sense of losing total control. On a higher level, it helps to teach the necessity of gaining control over the emotions so the emotional intensity will not distort one's natural energies.

Negative Condition: Fear of losing control; hysteria; pain with no apparent cause

Positive Outcome: Calm and centered in times of inner and outer turmoil; emotional balance

FIVE CORNERS *(low self-esteem, crushed)*

This Essence resolves low self-esteem, lack of confidence, and diminished love. It allows the life force to flow leaving a person feeling good and strong in themselves, and they feel their own love and beauty. In the negative mode, the person will appear crushed and "held in".

Negative Condition: Low self-esteem; dislike of self; crushed, held-in personality; clothing drab and colorless

Positive Outcome: Love and acceptance of self; a celebration of own beauty; joyousness

FLANNEL FLOWER *(discomfort with intimacy)*

This Essence is for people who are uncomfortable with emotional intimacy as well as physical contact and touching. They often have difficulty in maintaining their personal boundaries. It helps one to totally trust and express verbally their innermost feelings. It brings to both males and females a desire to and enjoyment in, expressing themselves physically. It is excellent for males allowing for gentleness, softness, and sensitivity in touching.

Negative Condition: Dislike of being touched; lack of sensitivity in males; uncomfortable with intimacy

Positive Outcome: Gentleness and sensitivity in touching; trust; openness; expression of feelings; joy in physical activity

FRESHWATER MANGROVE *(opens the heart to new experience)*

This Essence helps to release and heal mental prejudice, allowing the heart to open without prejudgment. It is for those who mentally reject or have already made up their mind about something without it ever being experienced. Often the seeds of this prejudice have been sown for a long time. In many cases, it is generational, as in the case of countries where religious prejudice is passed on and accepted by the young without question. This Essence has the potential to allow us to fully experience and be open on both a mental and heart level to new perceptual shifts and all the changes occurring at this time.

Negative Condition: Heart closed due to expectations or prejudices which have been taught, not personally experienced.

Positive Outcome: Openness to new experiences, people and perceptual shifts; healthy questioning of traditional standards and beliefs

FRINGED VIOLET *(protect and heal aura)*

This Essence is for treating damage to the aura where there has been shock, grief, or distress (e.g. from abuse or assault). This remedy maintains psychic protection and is excellent for people who are drained by others or those who unconsciously absorb the physical and emotional imbalances of others. It releases shock from the body. When used in combination with Flannel Flower or Wisteria it is beneficial for those who have suffered abuse.

Negative Condition: *Damage to aura; distress; lack of psychic protection*

Positive Outcome: *Removal of effects of recent or old distressing events; heals damage to aura; psychic protection*

GREEN ESSENCE *(harmonize yeast and mold)*

This Essence is not from flowers, but rather the stems and leaves of traditional, fresh, green herbs. It is used to harmonize any internal yeast, mold, and parasites to the same vibration as one's body. It should be taken orally for a minimum of two weeks, f,ve drops 3 times daily, five minutes before meals. It can also be used topically on the skin or internally as a douche.

Negative Condition: *Emotional distress associated with intestinal and skin disorders*

Positive Outcome: *Harmonizes the vibration of any yeast, mold, or parasite to one's own vibration; purifying*

GREEN SPIDER ORCHID *(past life phobias)*

This Essence is very much aligned with higher learnings, philosophies, and deeper insight. This Essence can assist in working with telepathy, to attune a person to be more receptive to not only other people but also other species and kingdoms. It is for people who are teaching spiritual matters and understandings, helping them to impart that knowledge. It also releases nightmares, terror, and phobias stemming from past lives.

Negative Condition: *Nightmares and phobias from past life experiences; intense negative reactions to the sight of blood*

Positive Outcome: *Telepathic communication; ability to withhold information until the timing is appropriate; attunement*

GREY SPIDER ORCHID *(extreme of psychic terror)*

This Essence helps to deal with extreme terror, especially terror experienced in life-threatening situations of psychic attack. It deals with panic and nightmares. This Essence will restore faith and trust.

Negative Condition: *Terror; fear of supernatural and psychic attack*

Positive Outcome: *Faith; calm; courage*

GYMEA LILY *(dominating, attention-seeking)*

This Essence is for excessive pride and arrogance and helps bring about humility. It is for reaching up to the energy of arrogance and transforming it to achieve great heights. It gives strength to those who are ahead of their peers and helps them to stay at the top. It is also very beneficial for people whose personalities are very intense or extroverted or those who are dominating, demanding, and very charismatic who usually get their way. It is also for people who like to be seen and noticed and who seek glamour and status.

Negative Condition: *Arrogant; attention-seeking; craving status and glamour; dominating and overriding personality*

Positive Outcome: *Humility; allowing others to express themselves and contribute; awareness, appreciation, and taking notice of others*

HIBBERTIA *(excessive self-discipline)*

This Essence is for people who are strict and regimented or even fanatical with themselves or for those who use their knowledge to gain an upper hand. They constantly devour information and philosophies purely to make themselves better people but often without truly integrating it. In the positive mode, these people will be accepting of themselves and their own innate knowledge and experiences, without wanting to be superior to others.

Negative Condition: *Fanatical about self-improvement; driven to acquire knowledge; excessive self- discipline; superiority*

Positive Outcome: *Content with own knowledge; acceptance; ownership and utilization of own knowledge*

ILLAWARRA FLAME TREE *(a deep sense of rejection)*

This Essence is for those who suffer from a great sense of rejection, or who feel "left out". this rejection is deeply felt and is very agonizing for the person. This Essence is also for self-rejection, or for a person feeling apprehensive about a new experience (e.g. parenthood, or where there is a fear of responsibility). This Essence will help a person take the first step. It is also beneficial for those whose numbers in numerology are 11, 22, or 33 – people who have usually chosen to do very important work in this life.

Negative Condition: *Overwhelming sense of rejection; fear of responsibility*

Positive Outcome: *Confidence; commitment; self-reliance; self-approval*

ISOPOGON *(learning from the past)*

This Essence is for people who live very much in their heads. They are dominated by their intellect and there is often a separation between their heart and head. This Essence, like Tall Yellow Top, connects one's emotions (heart) with their thoughts (head). It especially benefits those people who control through stubbornness. It enables the retrieval of long-forgotten skills and information.

Negative Condition: *Inability to learn from past experience; stubborn; controlling personality* **Positive Outcome:** *Ability to learn from past experience; retrieval of forgotten skills; relating without manipulating or controlling; ability to remember the past*

JACARANDA *(to be centered and decisive)*

This Essence is for people who dither, never completing things because they are constantly changing what they are doing.

Negative Condition: *Scattered; changeable; dithering; rushing*

Positive Outcome: *Decisiveness; quick-thinking; centered*

KANGAROO PAW *(unaware and socially inept)*

This Essence is for people who are "green" and socially inept. They do not know how to properly interact with other people. They can be very insensitive because they are so focused on themselves that they miss the cues and needs of other people around them. They can be very self-centered.

Negative Condition: *Gauche; unaware; insensitive; inept; clumsy*

Positive Outcome: *Kindness; sensitivity; savior faire; enjoyment of people; relaxed*

KAPOK BUSH *(apathetic and resigned)*

This Essence is for people who have a tendency to give up very easily, who are easily discouraged. It can also give people an overview of a plan or situation and then allow them to work it through sequentially and be able to bring it to fruition. It could even be for someone with a piece of technology or machinery, to assist them to understand how it works.

Negative Condition: *Apathy; resignation; discouraged; half-hearted*

Positive Outcome: *Willingness; application; "give it a 'go'"; persistence; perception*

LICHEN *(supports significant transitions)*

This Essence helps an individual to be aware of, look for and go to the Light at the moment of physical death. The alternative to the soul going through to the Light is to stay earthbound in the astral plane – what we commonly refer to as "a ghost". There is a great deal of darkness operating on the astral plane and it is certainly a level that the soul would be well-advised to move through quickly. A violent or sudden death can also result in the increased likelihood of the Spirit staying earthbound and the spraying of Lichen from an atomizer bottle would be of great benefit for these souls, helping them to see and go to the Light. Even where there is an unexpected sudden death (e.g. a car accident) the individual who dies in such an experience is fully aware at the level of their Higher Self, of what is about to happen and that they are going to pass over. Two weeks before such an event the etheric body starts to disengage and unravel from the physical body. Lichen assists the etheric and the physical bodies to separate in preparation for passing over.

Negative Condition: Not knowing to look for and move into the Light when passing over; earth bound in the astral plane

Positive Outcome: Eases one's transition into the Light; assists separation between the physical and etheric body; releases earthbound energies

LITTLE FLANNEL FLOWER (find joy, playfulness)

This Essence deals with the child aspect in us all. It addresses the expression of playfulness, being carefree and spontaneous joy. It is for people who regard life as a very somber and serious experience. It is also for children who tend to grow up much too quickly, who take on the troubles of the world and get old before their time. It helps children get in contact with their spirit guides.

Negative Condition: Denial of the "child" within; seriousness in children; grimness in adults

Positive Outcome: Carefree; playfulness; joyful

MACRO BUSH or MACROCARPA (endurance, inner-strength)

This Essence brings about renewed enthusiasm, endurance, and inner strength.

Negative Condition: Drained; jaded; worn-out

Positive Outcome: Enthusiasm; inner-strength; endurance

MINT BUSH (cope with spiritual emergence)

This Essence helps one cope with being tested to their limit. There is usually a great deal of confusion and one can have a sense that everything is too difficult and too much to deal with and resolve. These feelings can also arise during intense changes in your life – divorce, bankruptcy, severe illness or accidents, changing religious beliefs or affiliations.

Negative Condition: Perturbation; confusion; spiritual emergence; initial turmoil and void of spiritual initiation

Positive Outcome: Smooth spiritual initiation; clarity; calmness; ability to cope

MONGA WARATAH (empowerment, the strength of will)

This Essence can help a person find their own inner strength which enables them to reach out. It addresses the negative conditions of disempowerment of being overly needy; of feeling not strong enough; of feeling unable to do things alone; of always needing the strength and support of others; feeling choked or stifled in situations or relationships and feeling not able to strong enough to leave. This Essence very much addresses co-dependency as well as strengthening one's will. Consequently, it can be thought of when working with addictions. It gives you the belief and sense that you can break any dependency upon a behavior, substance, or person. It helps one to reclaim their spirit.

Negative Condition: Neediness; co-dependency; inability to do things alone; disempowerment; addictive personality

Positive Outcome: Strengthening of one's will; reclaiming of one's spirit; belief that one can break the dependency of any behavior, substance, or person; self-empowerment

MOUNTAIN DEVIL (anger and blocks to love)

This Essence helps one to deal with feelings of hatred, anger, jealousy, and the major blocks of expressing love. It is for people who tend to be suspicious of others. It helps to develop unconditional love and acceptance. It helps one to express anger in a healthy way and to develop sound boundaries which may open the way to forgiveness.

Negative Condition: Hatred; anger; holding of grudges; suspiciousness

Positive Outcome: Unconditional love; happiness; healthy boundaries; forgiveness

MULLA MULLA *(pain, fear of burns)*

This Essence is for personal recovery from the shattering experience of burns from heat or fire. It reduces the negative effects of fire and the sun's rays. IT is for those with a fear of fire or flames (often from a past life). If this fear is unconscious, it will often manifest in a lack of vitality, as if they wish to fade away. If a person presents with this picture they can, with appropriate counseling, reveal this fear of fire or hot objects.

Negative Condition: *Fear of flames and hot objects; distress associated with exposure to heat and sun*

Positive Outcome: *Reduces the effects of f,re and the sun; feeling comfortable with f,re and heat*

OLD MAN BANKSIA *(unenthusiastic and weary)*

This Essence is for people who are weary, frustrated and disheartened by setbacks. It helps to bring a spark into those people's lives who are heavy and slow-moving. They tend to be reliable, dependable people who steadily plod on, often hiding the weariness while battling on with unceasing effort.

Negative Condition: *Weary; phlegmatic personalities; disheartened; frustrated*

Positive Outcome: *Enjoyment of life; renews enthusiasm; interest in life*

PAW PAW *(absorbing new information)*

This Essence is for the assimilation and integration of new ideas and information, especially where there is a tendency to feel overwhelmed by the quantity of that information. It should be used when one is unable to solve a problem. It will activate the Higher Self, where we have the answers to all our problems. It will ease the burden of problems as it activates the intuitive processes to provide solutions.

Negative Condition: *Overwhelm; unable to resolve problems; burdened by decision*

Positive Outcome: *Improved access to Higher Self for problem-solving; assimilation of new ideas; calmness; clarity*

PEACH FLOWERED TEA TREE *(commitment, stability)*

This Essence is for people with extreme mood swings, hypochondriacal people, and those who have a fear of getting old. It can also be used for people who get enthusiastic and then, for no apparent reason, lose that enthusiasm. It is for those who do not "follow through" on their goals and convictions. Once the challenge goes, they become bored and lose interest. It will help develop stability, consistency, drive, and commitment.

Negative Condition: *Mood swings; lack of commitment to follow through on projects; easily bored; hypochondriacs*

Positive Outcome: *Ability to complete projects; personal stability; take responsibility for one's health*

PHILOTHECA *(accepting love)*

This Essence allows people to accept acknowledgment for their achievements and to "let in" love. They are often good listeners and generous, giving people. It allows shy people to speak of their plans and success.

Negative Condition: *Inability to accept acknowledgment; excessive generosity*

Positive Outcome: *Ability to receive love and acknowledgment; ability to let in praise*

PINK FLANNEL FLOWER *(gratitude, appreciation)*

This Essence is all about heart energy. It allows one to be in a state of gratitude for all aspects of their life and for what they are experiencing around them. It brings about an appreciation of and helps one take delight and pleasure in, the details and little things in life; to see and be aware of the blessings in every moment. It has been over forty years since this was last seen flowering, which explains why some Botanists and local people doubt its actual existence.

Negative Condition: Feeling and seeing life to be dull, flat, and lackluster; unappreciative; unhappy; taking for granted; unmindful

Positive Outcome: Gratitude; open-hearted; joie de vivre; appreciative; the lightness of being

PINK MULLA MULLA (deep healing and trust)

This Essence is for those who have suffered a deep spiritual wound long ago, often in their first incarnation, where they felt abandoned by Spirit which has led to a deep scar on the soul and psyche. It works on the outer causal bodies clearing sabotage (and fear of spiritual abandonment once more) that is stopping their spiritual growth. On an emotional level, Pink Mulla Mulla is for those who put out prickles to keep people away. They tend to be quite isolated and unable to resolve a hurt, wrong, or injustice which can be felt very deeply. This impinges on their attitude to those around them and can make them suspicious of people's motives, allowing them no rest. They are often on guard against people hurting them again, they may protect themselves by saying hurtful things to others. What they say to those around them does not always reflect how they really feel. It is merely a way of keeping people at a safe distance.

Negative Condition: Deep ancient wound on the psyche; an outer-guarded and prickly personal to prevent being hurt; keeps people at a distance

Positive Outcome: Deep Spiritual healing; trusting and opening up

RED GREVILLEA (become true to self)

This Essence is for people who feel stuck. It acts as a catalyst for those who know what they want to achieve but do not know how to go about it. It is for people who are too reliant on others. It promotes independence and boldness. This Essence is extremely effective though the changes may not be anticipated.

Negative Condition: Feeling stuck; oversensitive; affected by criticism and unpleasant people; too reliant on others

Positive Outcome: Boldness; strength to leave unpleasant situations; indifference to the judgment of others

RED HELMET ORCHID (resolving father issues)

This Essence helps a man bond to his child or children. It helps men to be aware to allocate quality family time. It is also for anyone with unresolved father issues, which can manifest as a recurrent, lifelong rebellious attitude to authority figures – police, bosses, etc.

Negative Condition: Rebelliousness; hot-headed; unresolved father issues; selfishness

Positive Outcome: Male-bonding; sensitivity; respect; consideration

RED LILY (live in the present)

This Essence is for spirituality and connection to God in a grounded and centered way, allowing a person to have a wholeness to their spirituality by also realizing the need to develop and maintain a balanced physical and emotional life.

Negative Condition: Vague; disconnected; split; lack of focus; daydreaming

Positive Outcome: Grounded; focused; living in the present; connection with life and God

RED SUVA FRANGIPANI (strength to cope)

This Essence addresses the great emotional intensity, difficulty, and hardship that people can go through when a relationship is ending, close to ending, or going through a very "rocky" period. It can also be taken for the enormous initial pain and sadness of the loss of a loved one. The person can be feeling greatly disturbed, not suicidal as in the case of Waratah, but torn apart by the event or situation.

Negative Condition: Initial grief, sadness, and upset of either a relationship at rock bottom or of the death of a loved one; emotional upheaval, turmoil, and rawness

Positive Outcome: Feeling calm and nurtured; inner peace and strength to cope

ROUGH BLUEBELL *(release malice, hurtfulness)*

This Essene helps people fully express the love vibration innate within them. It is for people who are very manipulative and for those who are deliberately malicious and use people, either subtly or openly. It can be for those who play the role of the martyr and like to have others obligated to them. They are aware of the needs of others but want love and affection for themselves and are not concerned about or unable to give it back.

Negative Condition: Deliberately hurtful, manipulative, exploitive, or malicious

Positive Outcome: Compassion; release of one's inherent love vibration; sensitivity

SHE OAK *(emotionally open to conceiving)*

This Essence is very beneficial in overcoming imbalances and bringing about a sense of well-being in females. It will benefit women who feel distressed about infertility. It removes those personal blocks that prevent conception. It can also be used in conjunction with Flannel Flower which will help remove karmic patterns hindering conception.

Negative Condition: Female imbalance; inability to conceive for non-physical reasons

Positive Outcome: Emotionally open to conceive; female balance

SILVER PRINCESS *(motivation, life's purpose)*

This Essence brings about awareness of one's life direction. Though it may not always reveal to a person their full life plan, it will aid people who are at crossroads, helping to show them what their next step is. It helps give them an understanding of that direction. This Essence is also excellent when one has reached an important goal and yet one is left feeling very flat, thinking "is this all there is". In this case, it gives one a glimpse or a sense of what is next and allows one to enjoy the journey whilst striving for the goal.

Negative Condition: Aimless; despondent; feeling flat; lack of direction

Positive Outcome: Motivation; direction; life purpose

SLENDER RICE FLOWER *(group harmony, co-operation)*

This Essence is for people who are racist, narrow-minded and lack humility. It can be used for group harmony and conflict resolution when individual egos get in that way. It allows for greater co-operation between people for the common good. This Essence has the ability to make an individual aware of the common divinity in all people.

Negative Condition: Prejudice; racism; narrow-mindedness; comparison with others

Positive Outcome: Humility; group harmony; co-operation; perception of beauty in others

SOUTHERN CROSS *(resolving victimhood)*

This Essence is for people who have a tendency to feel that they are a victim, that life has been hard on them. It helps people to understand that they create all the situations that happen to them in life and that they can change their situation by changing their thoughts.

Negative Condition: Victim mentality; complaining; bitter; martyrs; poverty consciousness

Positive Outcome: Personal power; taking responsibility; positiveness

SPINIFEX *(victim to illness)*

This Essence is the first Essence made from a grass species. It is for those who have a sense of being a victim to and having no control over illnesses, especially those with persistent and recurring symptoms.

Negative Condition: *Sense of being a victim to illness*

Positive Outcome: *Empowers one through an emotional understanding of illness*

STURT DESERT PEA *(deep emotional pain and hurt)*

This Essence is for deep hurts and sorrows. There are at least three Aboriginal legends connecting this flower to grief and sadness. This is one of the most powerful Essences and it can help the person bring about amazing changes in their life.

Negative Condition: *Emotional pain; deep hurt; sadness*

Positive Outcome: *Letting go; triggers healthy grieving; releases deep-held grief and sadness*

STURT DESERT ROSE *(guilt and remorse)*

This Essence is for guilt, including sexual guilt, which can be an emotional trigger for many sexual problems. It is also for following your own inner convictions and morality, helping you to follow through with what you know you have to do. If one is not true to themselves then there can often arise, as a consequence, feelings of regret or remorse. It can restore self-esteem that has been damaged by past actions you may have felt guilty about.

Negative Condition: *Guilt; regret and remorse; low self-esteem; easily led*

Positive Outcome: *Courage; conviction; true to self; integrity*

SUNDEW *(focused, present)*

This Essence is for people who are vague and indecisive and do not pay attention to detail. It is for those who tend to "split off" easily, especially when there is work to be done. This Essence will keep them focused on the present and reduces procrastination. It is for those who tend to be vague, dreamy, or drawn to drugs.

Negative Condition: *Vagueness; disconnectedness; split; indecisive; lack of focus; daydreaming*

Positive Outcome: *Attention to detail; grounded; focused; living in the present*

SUNSHINE WATTLE *(open to bright future)*

This Essence is for people who have had a difficult time in the past and who are stuck there They bring their negative experiences of the past into the present. Life is seen as being grim and full of struggle. When they look at life, they only see bleakness, hard times, and disappointment continuing into the future. In the positive mode, these people will see the beauty, joy, and excitement in the present and optimistically anticipate the future.

Negative Condition: *Stuck in the past; expectation of a grim future; struggle*

Positive Outcome: *Optimism; acceptance of the beauty and joy in the present; open to a bright future*

SYDNEY ROSE *(love and unity)*

This Essence helps a person to realize and to know on a deep heart-level and not merely an intellectual level...that there is no separation between us, that we are all one.

Negative Condition: *Feeling separated, deserted, unloved, or morbid*

Positive Outcome: *Realizing we are all one; feeling safe and at peace; heartfelt compassion; a sense of unity*

TALL MULLA MULLA *(for the socially ill at ease)*

This Essence is for people who are not at ease being with others. They prefer their own company and enjoy being alone but miss out on the emotional growth that interaction with others can bring. On an emotional level, there is not much "circulating with people" as it feels too troublesome and uncomfortable. They do not easily mix with others. They prefer to be alone where they know their own environment and can avoid confrontation with others. They will often go to any length to keep the peace even if it means agreeing to or saying things they don't believe. They do not breathe in life deeply for they prefer holding on to the familiar rather than being open to the new.

Negative Condition: *Ill at ease; sometimes fearful of circulating and mixing with others; loner; distressed by and avoids confrontation*

Positive Outcome: *Feeling relaxed and secure with other people; encourages social interaction*

TALL YELLOW TOP *(alienation and belonging)*

This Essence is for alienation. There is no feeling of connection or sense of belonging to family, workplace, country, self, etc. Often as a consequence of alienation the head, or intellect, takes over from the heart. As many people have been in this state for a long time, Tall Yellow Top will often need to be used for longer periods, sometimes for up to 6-8 weeks without a break. It is important when in this state to reach out to others for support.

Negative Condition: *Alienation; loneliness; isolation*

Positive Outcome: *Sense of belonging; acceptance of self and others; knowing that you are "home"; ability to reach out*

TURKEY BUSH *(creative expression)*

This Essence is all about creativity. It is for both the beginner and the artist. It allows a person to tune into their Higher Self and helps them to move through creative block and discouragement. This Essence brings about a desire to express and allows creativity to flow.

Negative Condition: *Creative block; disbelief in own creative ability*

Positive Outcome: *Inspired creativity; creative expression; focus; renews artistic confidence*

WARATAH *(black despair)*

This Essence is for the person who is going through the "black night of the soul" and is in utter despair. It gives them the strength and courage to cope with their crisis and will bring their survival skills to the forefront. This Essence will also enhance and amplify those skills. It is for emergencies and great challenges.

Negative Condition: *Despair; hopelessness; inability to respond to a crisis*

Positive Outcome: *Courage; tenacity; adaptability; strong faith; enhancement of survival skills*

WEDDING BUSH *(commitment, dedication)*

This Essence is excellent for commitment, whether in relationships, employment, the family, or personal goals. It can be of great benefit for a relationship when one or both individuals are uncertain if they wish to work through the issues their partner is bringing up to them. It can also be used for people who flit from one relationship to another or for when the initial attraction in the relationship diminishes.

Negative Condition: *Difficulty with commitment*

Positive Outcome: *Commitment to relationships; commitment to goals; dedication to life purpose*

WILD POTATO BUSH *(physically weighed down)*

This Essence is an excellent remedy for anyone feeling burdened or frustrated by any physical restriction or limitation with their body. This Essence brings about a sense of renewed enthusiasm, freedom, and the ability to move on in life. It is especially for those who feel heavy and need to step out of the old self, but who feel it is difficult to do so.

Negative Condition: *Weighed-down; feeling encumbered*

Positive Outcome: *Ability to move on in life; freedom; renews enthusiasm*

WISTERIA *(sensuality, gentleness)*

This Essence is for women who are uncomfortable with their sexuality. They may be unable to relax and enjoy sex, or afraid of physical intimacy and/or sensuality. It is especially beneficial for those who have had traumatic sexual experiences.

Negative Condition: *Feeling uncomfortable with sex; closed sexuality; macho male*

Positive Outcome: *Sexual enjoyment; enhanced sensuality; sexual openness; gentleness*

YELLOW COWSLIP ORCHID *(from critical to constructive)*

This Essence is about social order, group activity, and harmony. When out of balance there is excessive judgment and criticism.

Negative Condition: *Critical; judgmental; bureaucratic; nit-picking*

Positive Outcome: *Humanitarian concern; impartiality – stepping back from emotions; construction; a   keener sense of arbitration*

BACH FLOWER REMEDIES

Flowers in nature have the ability to affect our emotions in a positive manner. Different flower energies can actually remove our emotional pain and suffering, which over time could harm our health and impair our body's ability to heal. Dr. Edward Bach discovered this connection and when he died in 1936 made sure that his original system would be simple and easy to follow.

The Bach Flower Remedies work in harmony with herbs, homeopathy, and medications and are safe for everyone (including children, pregnant women, pets, the elderly, and even plants)

AGRIMONY

"The jovial, cheerful, humorous people who love peace and are distressed by argument or quarrel, to avoid which they will agree to give up much. Though generally they have troubles and are tormented and restless and worried in mind or in body, they hide their cares behind their humor and are considered very good friends to know. They often take alcohol or drugs in excess, to stimulate them and help themselves bear their trials with cheerfulness."—Dr. Edward Bach

Keywords: *Addiction, unhappy, anxiety, insomnia*

Human Indication: *Mental torment hidden behind a brave face. Appear care-free and humorous in order to mask anxieties and unhappiness.*

ASPEN

"Vague unknown fears for which there can be given no explanation, no reason. It is a terror that something awful is going to happen even though it is unclear what exactly. These vague inexplicable fears may haunt by night or day. Sufferers may often be afraid to tell their trouble to others." – Dr. Edward Bach

Keywords: *Fear, worries, unknown fears*

Human Indication: *Fears and worries of unknown origin.*

Pet Indication: *Vague or unaccountable fears. Appearing agitated for no apparent reason.*

BEECH

"For those who feel the need to see more good and beauty in all that surrounds them. And, although much appears to be wrong, to have the ability to see the good growing within. So as to be able to be more tolerant, lenient and understanding of the different way each individual and all things are working to their own perfection." —Dr. Edward Bach

Keywords: *Intolerance, critical, lack of compassion*

Human Indication: *When you need more tolerance toward other people.*

Animal/Pet indication: *Intolerance toward animals, people, events, and situations.*

CENTAURY

"Kind, quiet, gentle people who are over-anxious to serve others. They overtax their strength in their endeavors. Their wish so grows upon them that they become more servants than willing helpers. Their good nature leads them to do more than their own share of work, and in so doing they may neglect their own particular mission in life" — Dr. Edward Bach

Keywords: *Weak-willed, bullied, unable to say no, imposed on, lack energy, tired, timid, passive, quiet*

Human indication: *When you have a hard time saying NO and therefore easily get imposed on.*

CERATO

"Those who have not sufficient confidence in themselves to make their own decisions. They constantly seek advice from others, and are often misguided" **– Dr. Edward Bach**

Keywords: Confirmation, seeking advice, do not trust own wisdom or judgment

Human indication: *When you do not trust your own judgment in decision-making.*

CHERRY PLUM

"Fear of mind being over-strained, of reason giving away, of doing fearful and dreaded things, not wished and known wrong, yet there comes the thought and impulse to do them." **– Dr. Edward Bach**

Keywords: Fear of losing control, temper tantrum, breakdown, abusive, rage, explode **Human indication:** *When you are in deep despair and feel like you are going to "lose it."* **Animal/Pet indication:** *A loss of self-control, violent scratching*

CHESTNUT BUD

"For those who do not take full advantage of observation and experience, and who take a longer time than others to learn the lessons of daily life. Whereas one experience would be enough for some, such people find it necessary to have more, sometimes several, before the lesson is learned. Therefore, to their regret, they find themselves having to make the same error on different occasions when once would have been enough, or observation of others could have spared them even that one fault." **– Dr. Edward Bach**

Keywords: Learning, repeating mistakes

Human indication: *Keeps repeating the same mistake, doesn't learn from past mistakes.*

Animal/Pet indication: *Repeated unsuccessful behavior patterns, doesn't learn from past mistakes.*

CHICORY

"Those who are very mindful of the needs of others they tend to be over-full of care for children, relatives, friends, always finding something that should be put right. They are continually correcting what they consider wrong, and enjoy doing so. They desire that those for whom they care should be near them" **– Dr. Edward Bach Keywords:** *Possessive, over-protective, self-centered, critical, nagging, self-pity, easily offended, manipulating, demanding*

Human indication: *When you find yourself manipulating and controlling your loved ones.*

Animal/Pet indication: *Possessive in nature, very territorial, manipulating, loving to be in control.*

CLEMATIS

"Those who are dreamy, drowsy, not fully awake, no great interest in life. Quiet people, not really happy in their present circumstances, living more in the future than in the present; living in hopes of happier times when their ideals may come true. In illness, some make little or no effort to get well, and in certain cases may even look forward to death, in the hope of better times; or maybe, meeting again some beloved one whom they have lost." **– Dr. Edward Bach**

Keywords: Daydreaming, dreaminess, withdrawing, lack of concentration

Human indication: *When you have a tendency to live in your own dream world with little interest in the real world, accident-prone, daydreaming.*

Animal/Pet indication: *No apparent interest in the world around them; animals that sleep all the time, have trouble paying attention, or seem to live more in a dream than in the present.*

CRAB APPLE

"This is the remedy of cleansing. For those who feel as if they have something not quite clean about themselves. Often it is something of apparently little importance, in others, there may be a more serious disease that is almost disregarded compared to the one thing on which they concentrate. In both types, they are anxious to be free from the one particular thing which is greatest in their minds and which seems so essential to them that it should be cured. They become despondent if treatment fails. Being a cleanser, this remedy purifies wounds if the patient has reason to believe that some poison has entered which must be drawn out." – Dr. Edward Bach

Keywords: Cleansing, poor self-image, sense of not being clean, obsessive, poor self-image

Human indication: When you feel unclean or have a hard time accepting your own self-image.

Cleansing: Use externally on ringworm, rashes, and warts.

Animal/Pet indication: Obsessive cleanliness, fastidiousness; excessive grooming. Pets with rashes.

ELM

"Those who are doing good work, are following the calling of their life and who hope to do something of importance, and this often for the benefit of humanity. At times there may be periods of depression when they feel that the task they have undertaken is too difficult, and not within the power of a human being." – Dr.Edward Bach

Keywords: Depression overwhelmed by responsibilities, despondent, exhausted

Human indication: Feeling overwhelmed and depressed, there is too much to do, and you don't feel that you can do it all.

Animal/Pet indication: Overwhelmed by a sense of responsibility from a temporary circumstance, abandoning their litter.

GENTIAN

"Those who are easily discouraged. They may be progressing well in illness or in the affairs of their daily life, but any small delay or hindrance to progress causes doubt and soon disheartens them." – Dr. Edward Bach **Keywords:** Discouraged, depressed

Human indication: When you easily get discouraged when faced with difficulties.

Animal/Pet indication: Despondency due to a setback; e.g.; not going for a walk, as usual, creates lethargy and sadness.

GORSE

"Very great hopelessness, they have given up belief that more can be done for them. Under persuasion or to please others they may try different treatments, at the same time assuring those around that there is so little hope of relief." – Dr. Edward Bach

Keywords: Hopelessness, despair, pessimism

Human indication: When you have the feeling of extreme hopelessness and despair.

Animal/Pet indication: Feeling hopeless despair.

HEATHER

"Those who are always seeking the companionship of anyone who may be available, as they find it necessary to discuss their own affairs with others, no matter who it may be. They are very unhappy if they have to be alone for any length of time."
– Dr. Edward Bach

Keywords: Talkative, demand attention, dislike being alone, lonely

Human indication: Helps when you are preoccupied with your own ailments and problems.

Animal/pet indication: Overly concerned with companionship, very demanding of attention, constant barking.

HOLLY

"For those who are sometimes attacked by thoughts of such kind as jealousy, envy, revenge, suspicion. For the different forms of vexation. Within themselves they may suffer much, often when there is no real cause for their unhappiness." **—Dr. Edward Bach**

Keyword: *Envy, jealousy, hate, insecurity, suspicious, aggressive, needs compassion*

Human indication: *When you need to overcome the feeling of hate, envy, and jealousy.*

Animal/pet indication: *Jealousy of other animals or a new baby in the home. Angry growling, hissing, barking, snapping, or unprovoked attacks*

HONEYSUCKLE

"Those who live much in the past, perhaps a time of great happiness, or memories of a lost friend, or ambitions which have not come true. They do not expect further happiness such as they have had." **– Dr. Edward Bach**

Keyword: *Homesickness, nostalgia, bereavement*

Human indication: *For over-attachment to past memories good or bad, can't let go of the past, homesickness.*

Animal/pet indication: *Homesickness or over-attachment to the past. Loss of owner or home.*

HORNBEAM

"For those who feel that they have not sufficient strength, mentally or physically, to carry the burden of life placed upon them; the affairs of every day seem too much for them to accomplish, though they generally succeed in fulfilling their task. For those who believe that some part, of mind or body, needs to be strengthened before they can easily fulfill their work." **—Dr. Edward Bach**

Keyword: *Weariness, bores, tired, needs strength, overworked, procrastination, doubting own abilities*

Human indication: *For weariness, mental rather than physical, the "Monday morning" feeling with a sense of staleness and lack of variety in life.*

Animal/pet indication: *Lethargy or lack of enthusiasm to go anywhere, but once engaged in an activity or game is fully involved.*

IMPATIENS

"Those who are quick in thought and action and who wish all things to be done without hesitation or delay. When ill they are anxious for a hasty recovery. They find it very difficult to be patient with people who are slow as they consider it wrong and a waste of time, and they will Endeavour to make such people quicker in all ways. They often prefer to work and think alone, so that they can do everything at their own speed." **– Dr. Edward Bach**

Keyword: *Impatience, irritated, nervy, frustration, fidgety, accident-prone, hasty*

Human indication: *Suitable for people who are easily irritated and impatient. They speak and think quickly, and are energetic, but tense.*

Animal/pet indication: *Inpatient and seeming to have boundless energy, can't wait to go for a walk or rushes ahead.*

LARCH

"For those who do not consider themselves as good or capable as those around them, who expect failure, who feel that they will never be a success, and so do not venture or make a strong enough attempt to succeed." **–Dr. Edward Bach**

Keyword: *Lack of confidence, depressed, discouraged, feeling of inferiority*

Human indication: *When you need more self-confidence.*

Animal/pet indication: *Lack of self-confidence or avoiding situations where they have to perform.*

MIMULUS

"Fear of worldly things, illness, pain, accidents, poverty, of dark, of being alone, of misfortune. The fears of everyday life. These people quietly and secretly bear their dread; they do not freely speak of it to others." – Dr. Edward Bach

Keyword: *Fear, blushing, stammering, shyness, timid, sensitive, lack of courage*

Human indication: *Fear of known things such as fear of being alone, fear of spiders, fear of flying, or fear of the dark. Shyness is also a known fear.*

Animal/pet indication: *For fears: afraid of lightning, visits to the vet. May shake or shiver when confronted. Shy and timid animals.*

MUSTARD

"Those who are liable to times of gloom or even despair, as though a cold dark cloud overshadowed them and hid the light and the joy of life. It may not be possible to give any reason or explanation for such attacks. Under these conditions it is almost impossible to appear happy or cheerful." – Dr. Edward Bach

Keyword: *Depression, deep gloom for no reason*

Human indication: *When you feel depressed for no reason. Like a dark cloud that destroys normal cheerfulness.*

Animal/pet indication: *If your pet seems depressed for no reason.*

OAK

"For those who are struggling and fighting strongly to get well, or in connection with the affairs of their daily life. They will go on trying one thing after another, though their case may seem hopeless. They will fight on. They are discontented with themselves if illness interferes with their duties or helping others. They are brave people, fighting against great difficulties, without loss of hope of effort." – Dr. Edward Bach

Keyword: *Exhaustion, overwork, workaholic, fatigued, over-achiever*

Human Indication: *When you are exhausted, but keep struggling.*

Animal/Pet Indication: *If your pet keeps struggling although it is exhausted, never seem to quit.*

OLIVE

"Those who have suffered much mentally or physically and are so exhausted and weary that they feel they have no more strength to make any effort. Daily life is hard work for them, without pleasure." – Dr. Edward Bach

Keyword: *Lack of energy, fatigue, convalescence*

Human indication: *When you are exhausted with no reserves of strength or energy.*

Animal/pet indication: *Exhaustion, fatigue due to overwork: for working animals or those involved in racing, competitive events, or shows.*

PINE

"For those who blame themselves. Even when successful they think they could have done better, and are never satisfied with the decisions they make. Would this remedy help me to stop blaming myself for everything?" – Dr. Edward Bach

Keywords: *Guilt, self-reproach, humble, apologetic, shame, unworthy, undeserving*

Human indication: *When you feel guilt and self-reproach, not necessarily based on any actual wrong-doing but destroys the possibility of joy in living.*

Animal/pet indication: *If an animal feels shame or guilt for which something it cannot control.*

RED CHESTNUT

"For those who find it difficult not to be anxious for other people. Often they have ceased to worry about themselves, but for those of." – Dr. Edward Bach

Keywords: *Worried, over-concern, fear*

Human indication: *When you feel over-concerned and worried for others.*

ROCK ROSE

"The remedy of emergency for cases where there even appears no hope. In accident serious or sudden illness, or when the patient is very frightened or terrified, or if the conditions is serious enough to cause great fear to those around. If the patient is not conscious the lips may be moistened with the remedy." – Dr. Edward Bach

Keywords: *Frozen fear, terror*

Human indication: *When you feel terror, or after a nightmare. The feeling that you cannot react or move.*

Animal/pet indication: *Terror, panic-stricken: body trembling, cowers, or runs away. Deer in the headlight.*

ROCK WATER

"Those who are very strict in their way of living; they deny themselves many of the joys and pleasures of life because they consider it might interfere with their work. They are hard masters to themselves. They wish to be well and strong and active and will do anything which they believe will keep them so. They hope to be examples which will appeal to others who may then follow their ideas and be better as a result." – Dr. Edward Bach

Keywords: *Self-repression, self-denial, self-perfection, overwork, self-sacrificing, opinionated*

Human indication: *This is indicated when you are too strict and set too-high standards for yourself, to the point of self-domination and self-martyrdom.*

SCLERANTHUS

"Those who suffer much from being unable to decide between two things, the first one seeming more right than the other. They are usually quiet people, and bear their difficulty alone, as they are not inclined to discuss it with others." – Dr. Edward Bach

Keyword: *Indecision, imbalance, uncertainty, dizziness*

Human indication: *When you suffer from indecision, particularly when faced with two choices.*

Animal/pet indication: *Animals who can't make up their mind; any swinging behavior pattern (eats/doesn't, sleeps a lot/no sleep).*

STAR OF BETHLEHEM

"For those in great distress under conditions which for a time produce great unhappiness. The shock of serious news, the loss of someone dear, the fright following an accident, and such like. For those who for a time refuse to be consoled, this remedy brings comfort." – Dr. Edward Bach

Keywords: *Trauma, after effect of shock, post-traumatic stress*

Human indication: *For after-effects of trauma or traumatic experience.*

Animal/pet indication: *Abused, mistreated in the past. Trauma or shock.*

SWEET CHESTNUT

"For those moments which happen to some people when the anguish is so great as to seem to be unbearable. When the mind or body feels as if it had borne to the uttermost limit of its endurance, and that now it must give way. When it seems there is nothing but destruction and annihilation left to face." – Dr. Edward Bach

Keywords: Extreme mental anguish, hopeless despair, intense sorrow

Human indication: When you feel hopeless despair, and you feel intense sorrow and feel destroyed by it.

VERVAIN

"Those with fixed principles and ideas, which they are confident are right, and which they very rarely change. They have a great wish to convert all around them to their own views of life. They are strong of will and have much courage when they are convinced of those things that they wish to teach. In illness, they struggle on long after many would have given up their duties."

– Dr. Edward Bach

Keywords: Over-enthusiasm, hyper-active, fanatical, highly strung

Human indication: For people who are strong-willed and highly strung with minds that race ahead of events.

Animal/pet indication: Enthusiastic, always want to be involved, high strung.

VINE

"Very Capable people, certain of their own ability, confident of success. Being so assured, they think that it would be for the benefit of others if they could be persuaded to do things as they themselves do, or as they are certain is right. Even in illness, they will direct their attendants. They may be of great value in emergency." – Dr. Edward Bach

Keywords: Domineering, inflexible, very capable, gifted, bullying, aggressive

Human indication: For those who dominate others. They know better than everyone else and put others down.

Animal/pet indication: Authoritative, dominant even over their owners.

WALNUT

"For those who have definite ideals and ambitions in life and are fulfilling them, but on rare occasions are tempted to be led away from their own ideas, aims and work by the enthusiasm convictions or strong opinions of others. The remedy gives constancy and protection from outside influences." – Dr. Edward Bach

Keywords: Change, link breaker, menopause, puberty, moving, let go of the past, protection

Human indication: Protection from outside influences and energies. Helps you adjust to major changes.

Animal/pet indication: For any period of change.

WATER VIOLET

"For those who in health or illness like to be alone. Very quiet people, who move about without noise, are aloof, leave people alone and go their own way. Often clever and talented. Their peace and calmness is a blessing to those around them."

– Dr. Edward Bach

Keywords: Proud, aloof, lonely, anti-social, disdainful, condescending, self-reliant, private

Human indication: People who feel lonely because they have a tendency to appear proud and anti-social.

Animal/pet indication: Unfriendly, stand-offish, they do not invite or welcome cuddles, petting, or obvious affection.

WHITE CHESTNUT

"For those who cannot prevent thoughts, ideas, arguments which they do not desire from entering their minds. Usually at such times when the interest of the moment is not strong enough to keep the mind full. Thoughts that worry and still remain, or if for a time thrown out, will return. They seem to circle round and round and cause mental torture. The presence of such unpleasant thoughts drives out peace and interferes with being able to think only of the work or pleasure of the day." – *Dr. Edward Bach*

Keywords: Repeated unwanted thoughts, mental arguments, concentration, sleeplessness, insomnia.

Human Indication: When your mind is cluttered with thoughts or mental arguments. You may be unable to sleep because of the thoughts.

WILD OAT

"Those who have ambitions to do something of prominence in life, who wish to have much experience, and to enjoy all that which is possible for them, to take life to the full. Their difficulty is to determine what occupation to follow; as although their ambitions are strong, they have no calling which appeals to them above all others. This may cause delay and dissatisfaction."

– *Dr. Edward Bach*

Keywords: Cross-road in life, decision making, lack of clarity, drifting in life

Human indication: When you are uncertain of the correct path in life. Helpful when you need to make important decisions.

Animal/pet indication: Loss of sense of direction or purpose; especially good for working or show animals who are being retired.

WILD ROSE

"Those who without apparently sufficient reason become resigned to all that happens, and just glide through life, take it as it is, without any effort to improve things and find some joy. They have surrendered to the struggle of life without complaint."

– *Dr. Edward Bach*

Keywords: Apathy, resignation, lost motivation, lack of ambition

Human indication: For anyone who is resigned to an unpleasant situation whether illness, a monotonous life, or uncongenial work.

Animal/pet indication: Lack of energy, enthusiasm, submissive, and disinterested.

WILLOW

"For those who have suffered adversity or misfortune and find these difficult to accept, without complaint or resentment, as they judge life much by the success which it brings. They feel that they have not deserved so great a trial that it was unjust, and they become embittered. They often take less interest and are less active in those things of life which they had previously enjoyed." – *Dr. Edward Bach*

Keywords: Self-pity, resentment, short-changed, poor me, sulky, irritable, grumbling, bitterness, blame, complain

Human indication: When you feel resentment, self-pity, and bitterness. You would like to regain a sense of humor and proportion.

Animal/pet indication: Sulky, self-pity

RESCUE REMEDY

This is designed to help deal with immediate problems. Many people chose to carry this blend in their purse, at the office, in the car, or even in the diaper bag to be used at any time.

- **Impatiens:** *For those who act and think quickly, and have no patience for what they see as the slowness of others. They often prefer to work alone. Teaches empathy and understanding of and patience with others. We've found it very fast- acting in alleviating an impatient attitude and lowering stress.*
- **Star of Bethlehem:** *For trauma and shock, whether experienced recently or in the past. Teaches the ability to recover from traumas and to integrate them into the present life.*
- **Cherry Plum:** *For those who fear losing control of their thoughts and actions and doing things they know are bad for them or which they consider wrong. Teaches trust in one's spontaneous wisdom and the courage to follow one's path.*
- **Rock Rose:** *For situations in which one experiences panic or terror.*
- **Clematis:** *For those who find their lives unhappy and withdraw into fantasy worlds. They are ungrounded and indifferent to the details of everyday life. Teaches one to establish a bridge between the physical world and the world of ideas; may foster great creativity. Is also used to bring clarity and alertness to the present moment.*

BACH FLOWER REMEDIES

AGRIMONY Cannot see truth, avoid conflict. Try to keep true feelings hidden from self & others with feigned carefree, happy demeanor.	**ASPEN** Tormented by unpleasant ideas or vague anxieties & fears	**BEECH** Deep seated, unconscious intolerance, disguised as excessive sense of tolerance & empathy	**CENTAURY** Excessively cheerful, or obsequious. Allow themselves to be used too often.	**CERATO** Insecure, do not know how to do things. Constantly seek the advice and counsel of others.
CHERRY PLUM Those in danger of committing irrational acts, or of losing their reason.	**CHESTNUT BUD** For those with difficulty learning, who continually make the same mistakes.	**CHICORY** Greedy people who sacrifice themselves for others in order to cling to them and get affection.	**CLEMATIS** Susceptible to fantasies and daydreams, tend to lose their grip on reality.	**CRAB APPLE** Feel impure, or poisoned. This may be physically, or spiritually.
ELM For those who suddenly feel unable to carry out an important responsibility or mission.	**GENTIAN** For people of weak will and a tendency to be easily discouraged.	**GORSE** People without hope, serious illness with poor prognosis. Pessimism.	**HEATHER** Egocentric people, needing recognition, who cannot be alone, and speak constantly of themselves.	**HOLLY** Those inclined to behave in an unfriendly or aggressive manner.
HONEYSUCKLE For people who cannot let go of the past.	**HORNBEAM** The demands of everyday life are too difficult, even though they are capable of fulfilling them.	**IMPATIENS** Impatient, restless people. Always in a rush.	**LARCH** Lack of self confidence. Self denial, give up easily. Shyness, timidity.	**MIMULUS** Suffering firm vague, generalised fears & anxieties.
MUSTARD Those who fall into depression, bad moods or melancholia from time to time without any apparent reason.	**OAK** For people who cannot give up. Uncompromising, compulsive sense of obligation, ambition.	**OLIVE** Physical & emotional exhaustion. General weakness (heart) Spiritual exhaustion after great exertion or serious illness	**PINE** Suffering guilt, bad conscience. Self judgment/rejection. Bound to authority. Perfectionism.	**RED CHESTNUT** Worry for others, neurotic sympathy. Altruistic. Excessive caring.
ROCK ROSE Emergencies, panic, shock. Psychic shock, loss of presence of mind.	**ROCK WATER** Those too hard on themselves, martyr like. Lack of joy, self torment, fear of emotions.	**SCLERANTHUS** For difficulty making decisions. Inconsistent, unstable, unreliable.	**STAR of BETHLEHEM** Those without the strength to bear unhappy situations. Devastating situations. Unprocessed trauma, physical or psychic.	**SWEET CHESTNUT** Total despair, on the verge of a total breakdown. Extreme depression. (Seldom needed in daily life)
VERVAIN Those trying to burden others with their convictions, missionary zeal. Pushy, one-sided.	**VINE** Self confident, intolerant. Dominant, superior.	**WALNUT** Easily influenced, lack inner stability.	**WATER VIOLET** Loners who have problems with human contact. Shy, reserved, unapproachable.	**WHITE CHESTNUT** Tyrannised by unpleasant thoughts. Sleepless, wired, headaches from stress, jumbled thoughts.
WILD OAT Seeking meaningful action, unsure how to achieve it. Discontented, frustrated, alienated.	**WILD ROSE** Resignation, apathy, convalescence. Can't get active, motivated.	**WILLOW** Disappointed, bitter, offended. Resentful, need revenge.	**RESCUE REMEDY** Cherry plum, Clematis, Impatiens, Rock Rose, Star of Bethlehem. Any emergency; calms, stabilises, heals.	

SCHUESSLER SALTS

A 19th-century German doctor named Dr. Wilhelm Heinrich Schuessler discovered that several mineral salts had notable health benefits; Dr. Schuessler developed these mineral salts homeopathically for assimilation by the cells of the body. This homeopathic healing method of cell salts is based on twelve basic remedies used for biochemical treatments.

No. 1 CALCIUM FLUORATUM *(Connective tissue, skin, joints)*

No. 2 CALCIUM PHOSPHATE *(Bones and teeth)*

No. 3 IRON PHOSPHATE *(Immune system)*

No. 4 POTASSIUM CHLORIDE *(Mucous membranes)*

No. 5 POTASSIUM PHOSPHATE *(Nervous system)*

No. 6 POTASSIUM SULPHATE *(Metabolism)*

No. 7 MAGNESIUM PHOSPHATE *(Muscles)*

No. 8 SODIUM CHLORIDE *(Water regulation)*

No. 9 SODIUM PHOSPHATE *(Metabolism)*

No. 10 SODIUM SULPHATE *(Purification)*

No. 11 SILICA *(Connective tissue, skin, hair)*

No. 12 CALCIUM SULPHATE *(Joints, pus)*

No. 13 POTASSIUM ARSENITE *(Skin, vitality)*

No. 14 POTASSIUM BROMIDE *(Nervous system, skin)*

No. 15 POTASSIUM IODIDE *(Sign gland)*

No. 16 LITHIUM CHLORIDE *(Rheumatism, nerves)*

No. 17 MANGANESE SULPHATE *(Iron System)*

No. 18 CALCIUM SULPHIDE *(Vitality, body-weight)*

No. 19 COPPER ARSENITE *(Digestive system, kidneys)*

No. 20 POTASSIUM ALUMINUM SULFURICUM *(Digestive system, nervous system)*

No. 21 ZINC CHLORIDE *(Metabolism, womb, nerves)*

No. 22 CALCIUM CARBONATE *(Vitality, Anti-Aging)*

No. 23 SODIUM BICARBONATE *(Purif,cation, Body acid balance)*

No. 24 ARSENIC IODIDE *(Skin, allergies)*

No. 25 AURUM CHLORATUM NATRONATUM *(Day and night rhythm, female reproductive organs)*

No. 26 SELENIUM *(Liver, blood vessels)*

No. 27 POTASSIUM DICHROMATE *(Blood, sugar metabolism)*

Description	Body Parts	Function	Symptoms
LC FLUOR 6X lcarea Fluorica, HPUS	Bones, elastic tissues, veins, arteries, teeth, joints	Gives tissues the quality of elasticity, preserves contractile power of elastic tissue.	Cracks in the skin, loss of elasticity, relaxed condition of the veins and arteries, piles, sluggish circulation, loose teeth.
LC PHOS 6X lcarea Phosphoricum, US	Bones, muscles, nerves, brain, connective tissues, teeth	Aids normal growth and development, restores tone and strength, aids digestion, aids bone and teeth formation.	Anemic state of young girls, blood coagulation problems, blood poverty, imperfect circulation, bone weakness, rickets.
LC SULPH 6X lcarea Sulphurica, HPUS	Blood, skin	Blood purifier and healer that removes waste products from the blood.	Pimples, sore throat, cold, all conditions arising from impurities in the blood.
ERRUM PHOS 6X rrum Phosphoricum, HPUS	Muscles, nerves, hair, blood vessels, arteries, red blood cells	First aid, oxygen carrier, supplementary remedy.	Congestion, inflammatory pain, high temperature, quickened pulse, lack of red blood corpuscles.
LI MUR 6X li Muriaticum, HPUS	Muscles, blood, saliva	Treats burns, aids digestions, cleanses and purifies the blood.	Sluggish conditions, catarrhs, sore throat, glandular swelling, white colored tongue, light colored stools, coughs, and colds.
LI PHOS 6X li Phosphoricum, HPUS	Muscles, nerves, skin	Nerve nutrient, aids breathing, contributes to a contented disposition, sharpens mental faculties.	Nervous headaches, lack of pep, ill humor, skin ailments, sleeplessness, depression, timidity, tantrums
LI SULPH 6X li Sulphuricum, HPUS	Skin, intestine, hair, stomach, tissue cells	Oxygen carrier, antifriction, maintains hair, benefits perspiration and respiration.	Boxed in feeling, intestinal disorders, stomach catarrh, inflammatory conditions, eruptions on the skin and scalp with scaling, shifting pains.
AG PHOS 6X agnesia Phosphoricum, PUS	Muscles, nerves, bones	Anti-spasmodic, benefits the nervous system, helps ensure rhythmic movement of muscular tissue.	Menstrual pains, stomach cramps, flatulence, neuralgia, sciatica, headaches with darting stabs of pain, cramps, muscular twitching.
AT MUR 6X atrum Muriaticum HPUS	Cartilage, mucus cells, glands	Water distributor, aids nutrition and glandular activity, aids cell division and normal growth, aids digestion.	Low spirits, headaches with constipation, heartburn, tooth ache, hay fever, craving for salt and salty foods, weak eyes
AT PHOS 6X atrum Phosphoricum PUS	Nerves, muscles, joints, digestive organs	Acid neutralizer, aids in the assimilation of fats and other nutrients.	Stiffness and swelling of the joints, acidic blood conditions, rheumatism, lumbago, worms, golden-yellow coating at root of tongue
AT SULPH 6X atrum Sulphuricum, HPUS	Liver, digestive system	Eliminates excess water, ensures adequate bile, removes poison-charged fluids, treats rheumatic ailments.	Influenza, humid asthma, malaria, liver ailments, brownish green coating of the tongue, bitter taste in mouth
LICA 6X licea, HPUS	Connective tissues, skin	Cleanser and eliminator, initiates the healing process, insulator of the nerves, restores the activity of the skin.	Smelly feet and arm pits, pus formation, abscesses, boils, tonsillitis, brittle nails, stomach pains.

VITAL SUBSTANCES

Healy Vital Substances Frequency Database:

L-ALANINE

Supports muscle enhancement and boosts energy. Regulates blood sugar. Supports the immune system and prostate.

L-ARGININE

Relaxes blood vessels and may help with erectile dysfunction. Lowers blood pressure. Supports endothelium health which may reduce the chance of heart attack or stroke.

L-ASPARAGINE

Supports brain development and function. Supports liver function. Regulates mood and the central nervous system.

L-CARNITINE

Supports muscle repair and regulates muscle pain. Use is effective in the following conditions: serious kidney disease, hyperthyroidism, male infertility, and myocardiditis (inflammation of the heart). Reduces memory issues in elderly people. Supports heart health. Supports weight loss and fat burning.

L-CYSTEINE

Antiaging properties. Supports immune function. Promotes detoxification from drug reactions and toxic chemicals. Increases male fertility. Balances blood sugar levels. Supports digestive health.
Relieves symptoms of respiratory conditions. Helps to treat psychiatric disorders as well as addictions. Other uses include acne, angina, asthma, emphysema, colon cancer, and lung cancer.

L-GLUTAMINE

A building block of protein. Used for weight loss, fat burning, and building muscle. Treats leaky gut syndrome. Improves gastrointestinal issues such as irritable bowel syndrome (IBS), Crohn's disease, ulcerative colitis, diverticulosis, and diverticulitis. Boosts brain health. Decreases muscle wasting. Improves athletic performance and exercise recovery. Suppresses insulin levels and stabilizes blood glucose.

GLUTAMIC ACID

Improves memory and focus. Boosts the immune system. Supports prostate health. Detoxes the body. Improves athletic performance. Supports digestive health.

GLUTAMATE

Acts as an important neurotransmitter in the brain. Supports growth and development of the brain. Supports cognitive functions, including learning and memory. Supports the "gut-brain connection". Helps with bone formation and muscle tissue repair.

L-GLYCINE

Helps build lean muscle mass. Prevents muscle wasting. Supports the production of human growth hormone. Boosts mental performance and memory. Helps to prevent ischemic strokes and seizures. Protects skin from signs of aging or cellular mutations. Protects collagen in joints and reduces joint pain. Supports flexibility and range of motion. Regulates blood sugar. Improves sleep. Reduces inflammation. Supports digestive health. Reduces allergic and autoimmune reactions.
Supports production of red blood cells. Helps control symptoms of mental disorders.

L-HISTIDINE

Supports the growth and creation of blood cells and tissue repair. Helps to maintain the protective covering over nerve cells (myelin sheath). The body metabolizes histidine into histamine, which is crucial for immunity, reproductive health, and digestion. Studies show that it may also lower BMI and insulin resistance in obese women and women with metabolic syndrome. Deficiency can cause anemia, and low blood levels appear to be more common among people with arthritis and kidney disease.

L-ISOLEUCINE

Lowers glucose. Decreases muscle damage and soreness. Reduces fatigue and boosts performance.

L-LEUCINE

Helps regulate blood sugar levels and aids the growth and repair of muscle and bone. It is also necessary for wound healing and the production of growth hormones. Deficiency can lead to skin rashes, hair loss, and fatigue.

L-LYSINE

Builds muscle; maintains bone strength, aids in recovery from injury or surgery, regulates hormones, antibodies, and enzymes. Possible antiviral effects.

L-METHIONINE

Along with cysteine, methionine supports the health and flexibility of skin, and hair, and the strength of nails. Supports proper absorption of selenium and zinc as well as the removal of heavy metals like lead and mercury.

L-ORNITHINE

Supports muscle strength and health. Supports liver detoxification by assisting with eliminating extra nitrogen and other waste such as ammonia. Stimulates liver tissue regeneration.

L-PHENYLALANINE

Used to treat vitiligo. Produces dopamine. Supports learning, memory, and emotion. May reduce symptoms of depression. May aid in the treatment of Parkinson's disease. Relieves chronic pain. May promote weight loss.

L-PROLINE

Helps to heal wounds and repair skin. Supports digestive health. Helps to prevent joint pain. Supports the cardiovascular system. Supports healthy metabolism and fights inflammation. Supports toe formation of new collagen. Naturally prevents or treats cellulite. Treats leaky gut syndrome.

L-PYRROLYSINE

The largest naturally occurring amino acid.

L-SELENOCYSTEINE

Supports heavy metal removal. Boosts immunity. Supports healthy gut.

L-SELENOMETHIONINE

Supports healthy thyroid gland function, reproduction, DNA production, and protecting the body from infection. Supports healthy heart function. Supports cognitive function.

L-SERINE

Improves brain function. Fights fibromyalgia. Helps to relieve stress. Improves sleep. Boosts immune function.

L-TAURINE

Helps to maintain proper hydration and electrolyte balance in your cells. Helps to form bile salts for digestion. Regulates minerals such as calcium within cells. Supports the central nervous system and eyes. Regulates immune system and antioxidant function.

L-THREONINE

Supports healthy skin and teeth; is a component of tooth enamel, collagen, and elastin. Helps to aid fat metabolism and may benefit people with indigestion, anxiety, and mild depression.

L-TRYPTOPHANE

Produces melatonin in the brain (pineal gland), the gut, the retina, and immune cells. Improves sleep quality and helps with insomnia. May improve obstructive sleep apnea. Helps with PMS. Assists with smoking cessation. May reduce symptoms of depression. May reduce manic symptoms. May reduce appetite. Used for dementia. Increases exercise performance, likely due to increased pain tolerance.

L-TYROSINE

May boost cognition and alertness under stress or sleep deprivation. May improve mood. May increase thyroid hormones. May help with fibromyalgia. Used for patients with narcolepsy.
Reduces addiction and substance withdrawal. May support weight loss.

L-VALINE

Essential for mental focus, muscle coordination, and emotional calm. Valine supplements are often used for muscle growth, tissue repair, and energy. Deficiency may cause insomnia and reduced mental function.

ALPHA-LINOLENIC ACID

Lowers cholesterol. Anti-asthmatic properties. Anti-inflammatory effects. Protection against breast cancer. Supports bone health. Benefits for pregnant women including a longer duration of gestation and greater birth weight.

LINOLEIC ACID

Supports heart health. Supports healthy brain function. Supports skin and hair health. Supports reproductive health. Boosts immune function. Protects bone density.

OMEGA-3 FATTY ACIDS

Reduces symptoms of depression and anxiety. Supports eye health and can reduce the risk of macular degeneration. Can promote brain health during pregnancy and early life. Supports heart health. Can reduce symptoms of ADHD in children. Can reduce symptoms of Metabolic Syndrome. Anti-inflammatory. Can fight autoimmune diseases, including type-1 diabetes, autoimmune diabetes, multiple sclerosis, lupus, rheumatoid arthritis, ulcerative colitis, Crohn's disease, and psoriasis. Can improve mental disorders. Can fight age-related mental decline and Alzheimer's disease. May help prevent cancer. Can reduce asthma in children. Can reduce fat in your liver. May improve bone and joint health. Can alleviate menstrual pain. May improve sleep. Supports healthy skin.

MYRISTIC ACID

Used in the fragrance and beauty industry.

PALMITIC ACID

Supports cellular functions. Helps to heal skin issues including rash, irritation and redness, dryness, and insect bites.

GAMMA-LINOLENIC ACID

Anti-inflammatory. Fights cell damage and regulates pain as part of the healing process. Prevents or treats a variety of health conditions, including asthma; atherosclerosis; cancer; diabetic neuropathy; eczema; chronic fatigue syndrome; depression; high-cholesterol; menopause symptoms; metabolic syndrome; psoriasis; and rheumatoid arthritis.

LAURIC ACID

Strong antimicrobial and antiviral properties; helps to treat or prevent infections, viruses, digestive disorders, and chronic disease. Positive outcomes for treating herpes simplex virus (HSV), chronic yeast infections, and HIV/AIDS and has been shown to kill staphylococcus Aureus. Also controls infections like bronchitis, candida virus, sexually transmitted diseases like gonorrhea, genital warts caused by human papillomavirus (HPS) or chlamydia, and intestinal infections caused by parasites. Helps fight antibiotic resistance. Supports heart health. Supports healthy skin and fights acne. Correlated with health and longevity in traditional populations.

OMEGA-6 FATTY ACIDS

May reduce symptoms of nerve pain in people with diabetic neuropathy. May reduce symptoms of Rheumatoid arthritis and assist with related joint pain. May reduce symptoms of ADHD. Reduces blood pressure and supports heart health. Supports bone health.

OLEIC ACID

Lowers total cholesterol. Decreases blood pressure. Boosts mood and energy. Improves cognition. Anti-inflammatory properties. Improves response to insulin. May decrease obesity. Anti-aging benefits for your skin.

EICOSAPENTAENOIC ACID

Lowers ADHD symptoms. Reduces symptoms of depression. Supports heart health. Reduces symptoms and inflammation caused by rheumatoid arthritis. Reduces hot flashes. Reduces menstrual cramping and pain. Reduces discomfort and sensitivity to cold for people with Raynaud syndrome. Reduces joint pain and fatigue from lupus. Positive effects have also been reported on kidney and lung disease, type-2 diabetes, anorexia nervosa, Crohn's disease, burns, osteoporosis, and early stages of colorectal cancer.

DOCOSAHEXAENOIC ACID

Reduces heart disease risk. May improve ADHD. Reduces the risk of early preterm births. Anti- inflammatory properties that may reduce the risk of chronic diseases that are common with age, such as heart and gum disease, and improve autoimmune conditions like rheumatoid arthritis, which causes joint pain. Supports muscle recovery after exercise. Supports eye health and may specifically improve dry eyes and diabetic eye disease (retinopathy). Known to lower the risk of several cancers, including colorectal, pancreatic, breast, and prostate. May help prevent or slow Alzheimer's disease. Lowers blood pressure and supports circulation. Aids normal brain and eye development in babies. Supports men's reproductive health. May reduce symptoms of depression.

DIHOMO-GAMMA-LINOLENIC ACID

Anti-inflammatory. Fights cell damage and regulates pain as part of the healing process. Prevents or treats a variety of health conditions, including asthma; atherosclerosis; cancer; diabetic neuropathy; eczema; chronic fatigue syndrome; depression; high-cholesterol; menopause symptoms; metabolic syndrome; psoriasis; and rheumatoid arthritis.

ARACHIDONIC ACID

Improves intelligence in early neurological development. Shown to lower symptoms and slow progression of Alzheimer's disease. Aids in the development of infants. Supports muscle health, liver health, and brain health. Treats parasites. Regulates glucose.

BORON

Relieves menstrual pain. Aids in wound healing. Supports bone health and helps to prevent arthritis. Enhances testosterone levels. Lowers plasma lipid levels. Can reduce fungal infections. Improves cognition.

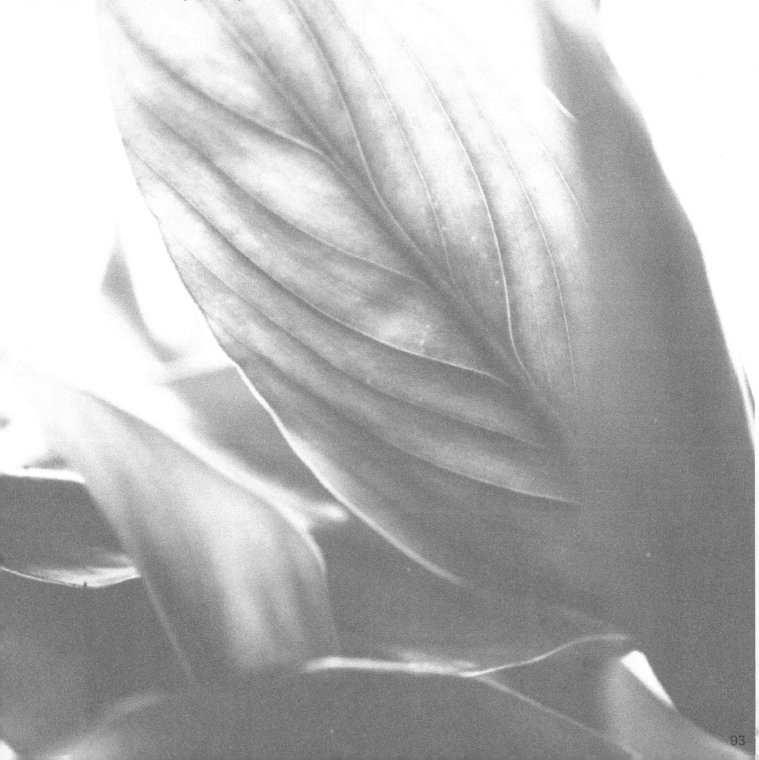

Video References

 Healy for Beginners

 Resonance Analysis Scan

 Aura Analysis

 Coaching Analysis

 Healy Q&A with Brid Hanlon

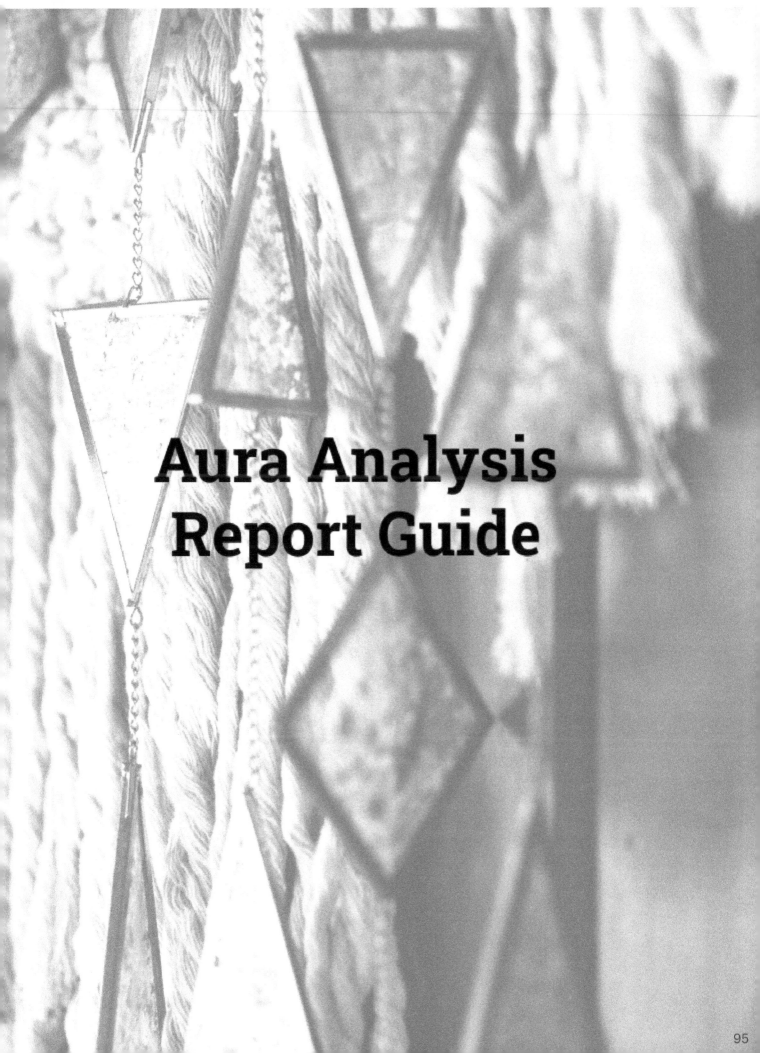

Aura Analysis
Report Guide

Aura Analysis Guidance

ENERGY READING COLOR SCALE

CHAKRA COLOR RESULT:	MEANING:
Same Chakra Color	The **energy is harmonized** with the chakra. **Reading is positive** in nature.
Partially contains Chakra Color	**Harmonization is already in progress**. Reading is **relatively positive**.
Other Chakra Color	Energy is **not harmonized** with the chakras. Identified chakra source is indication of potential issue.
Turquoise	Signifies a **readiness for harmonization**. Reading is **encouraging**.
Black	A **theme of the chakra is denied**. The invitation is **self reflection to identify what you are denying or resistin**
White	A **theme of the chakra is avoided**. The invitation is **self reflection to identify what you are avoiding or igno**

INTENSITY LEVEL

88% | 4 | LM XXIV - 11.19.2022 05:31:26

Intensity level refers to:
- The level of presence of that specified energy in that chakra center
- The level of effort to transmute/release the energy blockage

(10) Substantial work to be done
Prioritize the topic revealed.

(5) Moderate effort to remedy

(1) Effortless and quickly remedied

RELEVANCE LEVEL

88% | 4 | LM XXIV - 11.19.2022 05:31:26

Relevance level refers to:
- How relevant and how important it is that this energy center is balanced right now

Include high negative relevancies

Start analysis

Include high negative relevancies means:
- Issues that the Healy scan finds that are present in your energy field however, they are not currently active in your life

POTENCY LEVEL

Potency level refers to the following:
- Location of the energy in the subtle anatomy
- The energy is manifesting and/or originating within these specific areas

88% | 4 | LM XXIV - 11.19.2022 05:31:26

LM	**MENTAL & SPIRITUAL** - Based on an erroneous belief system	**1 - 60** **I - LX**	Incoherence in **Actions**	**1E6**	**Karmic** - originates from another incarnation
C	**EMOTIONAL** - Emotional charge not expressed	**100 - 400** **C - CD**	Incoherence in **Thought Pattern**	**1E12**	**Family** – originates from parents
		1000 - 2000 **M - MM**	Incoherence in the chosen **Lifestyle**	**1E24**	**Family** – originates from grandpare
D	**PHYSICAL** - Deeply rooted and repressed for a long period of time	**10 000 - 100 000**	Incoherence in a **Life Theme**	**1E36**	**Ancestral** – originates from ancesto

Coaching Analysis
Report Guide

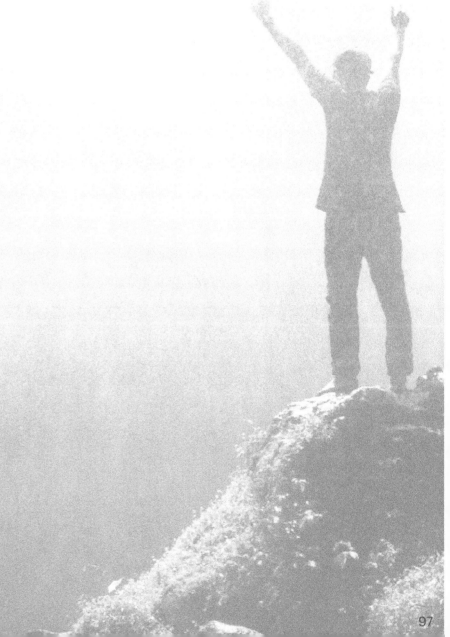

Coaching Analysis Chart

HEALY LIST OF POTENCIES
TIMEWAVER HOMEOPATHIC CODES

D = PHYSICAL	C = MENTAL / EMOTIONAL	LM = SPIRITUAL
WRONG ACTING		
D 1	C 1	LM I
D 2	C 2	LM II
D 3	C 3	LM III
D 4	C 4	LM IV
D 6	C 6	LM VI
D 8	C 8	LM VIII
D 12	C 12	LM XII
D 15	C 15	LM XV
D 18	C 18	LM XVIII
D 23	C 23	LM XXIII
D 24	C 24	LM XXIV
D 30	C 30	LM XXX
D 60	C 60	LM LX
WRONG THINKING		
D 100	C 100	LM C
D 200	C 200	LM CC
D 400	C 400	LM CD
WRONG LIFESTYLE / LACKING TRUST		
D 1000	C 1000	LM M
D 2000	C 2000	LM MM
LIFE THEME		
D 10,000	C 10,000	LM 10,000
D 50,000	C 50,000	LM 50,000
D 100,000	C 100,000	LM 100,000
KARMIC D 1E6	C 1E6	LM 1E6
PARENTAL D 1E12	C 1E12	LM 1E12
GRANDPARENTS D 1E24	C 1E24	LM 1E24
ANCESTORS D 1E36	C 1E36	LM 1E36

WRONG ACTING
• Currently present in our lives
• A phase or seasonal transition
• Misaligned decisions/choices with actions

WRONG THINKING
• Negative future projections
• Feelings of worry, fear, aniexty, guilt
• Misperceptions or incorrect interpretations

WRONG LIFESTYLE / LACKING TRUST
• Poor lifestyle habits
• Substance abuse (alcohol, drugs, food, shopping, addictions)
• Negative influences (social media, television, family, friends, colleagues)
• Sedentary lifestyle (lack of movement, connection with nature, not grounded, de-pressed emotions , lack of engagement/socializing)

LIFE THEME
• Common thread present in life
• Programming - mentally, emotionally, physically
• Deep unconscious beliefs
• Culturally instilled ideas and belief systems
• Disconnection to Self/ Source. Separation.

My Healy Journey

JOURNALING SUGGESTIONS

Reflection

Take a moment to tune in and capture what you are feeling emotional, sensing physically, as well as the quality of your thoughts.

After running a program, notice any shifts in your emotions, physical sensations and/or symptoms, thoughts, as well as your energy level and capture it.

Then, reflecting on your current state, recall your state prior to running the prog and notice any messages you received or shifts you experienced.

Perspective

Without any judgement, notice your perspective and what resonates with you an journal what that currently is.

After running a scan, journal any information that you became conscious of and potentially shifted your view.

Take Aways

After running a scan and/or program what insights did you come to see?
Did you learn anything new about yourself?
Did you notice if any specific results seemed to not resonate with you?
What results did resonate with you?
Were there any results that did not resonate with you that later did make sense were relevant?

Lessons

List any lessons you have experienced during your journey with Healy.
What changes and shifts have you experienced or are experiencing?
Have you experienced any challenges that resulted in breakthroughs?

Self Love

How has using Healy allowed you to connect deeper with yourself?
In what ways has using Healy taught you to trust more?
Have you experienced any changes in your intuition?
Have you experienced greater appreciation for yourself, your life and others?
If so, capture what you are grateful for and how Healy has been a part of your self-love journey.

Free Style

Express yourself in any way you feel called to.

Printed in the USA
CPSIA information can be obtained
at www.ICGtesting.com
LVHW061252211123
764112LV00014B/680